What People Are Saying About
Breast Cancer Smoothies

"Daniella is one of my favorite health experts and does superb work. I couldn't recommend her book more highly. Read this book and follow her advice. It's that simple!"

—**Anahad O'Connor**, *The New York Times*

"Research consistently shows us that following a whole foods, plant-based diet can be integral in cancer prevention and recovery. *Breast Cancer Smoothies* provides accessible recipes backed by academic research, plus important nutritional guidance. Whether you have been affected by breast cancer or not, Daniella's smoothies are an easy, delicious way to transform your health!"

—**Dr. Neal Barnard**, founding president of
the Physician's Committee for Responsible Medicine

"Delicious culinary medicine has never been easier, faster, or backed by better science. Daniella's delicious, inventive, real food recipes will help you fight fatigue and boost your energy level if you have or want to prevent breast cancer . . . and want to know how to use your kitchen medicine cabinet and blender to do it."

—**John La Puma, M.D.**, ChefMD®, two-time *New York Times*
bestselling author and founder of Chef Clinic®

"The bodies of cancer patients are starving for beneficial, life-supporting, degeneration-reversing, health-stimulating, nutrients to optimize immune function and unleash the body's potential for good health. The good news is that Nature is rich and bountiful with everything the body needs—and provides it in an amazing and delightful variety of foods and tastes. Daniella Chace has provided a road map to this healing treasure trove that is simple, easy and fun to follow. Who knew that getting healthy could taste so good?"

—**William Wolcott**, author of *The Metabolic Typing Diet*

"Smoothies pack a punch when it comes to nutrients. This collection of delicious and nutritious smoothies features ingredients that have been scientifically studied to be active against breast cancer. This takes out the guess work for women concerned about their breast cancer risk. All that is left is the task of chopping, blending, and enjoying! This book is a must-have for women who want to take their diet to the next level of health optimization."

—**Dr. Lise Alschuler, ND, FABNO**, coauthor, *Definitive Guide to Cancer* and *Definitive Guide to Thriving After Cancer*

"This book is full of flavorful smoothies with healing effects for breast cancer. Daniella helps the reader organize their kitchen and prepare foods so that blending smoothies is easy and convenient. She describes what each food does for the body and lists reference articles that discuss their medicinal effects. Daniella brings a great knowledge of oncology nutrition and smoothie making together for patients in this complete guide that provides help for anyone who wants to prevent or heal from breast cancer."

—**Dr. Leah McNeill, ND**, director of Ohana Wellness Center, Bellevue, WA

BREAST CANCER SMOOTHIES

100 Delicious, Research-Based Recipes for Prevention and Recovery

DANIELLA CHACE, MS, CN

From the bestselling author of
More Smoothies for Life and *Turning Off Breast Cancer*

Health Communications, Inc.
Deerfield Beach, Florida

www.hcibooks.com

**Library of Congress Cataloging-in-Publication Data
is available through the Library of Congress**

© 2016 Daniella Chace, MS, CN

ISBN-13: 978-07573-1939-6 (Paperback)
ISBN-10: 07573-1939-4 (Paperback)
ISBN-13: 978-07573-1940-2 (ePub)
ISBN-10: 07573-1940-8 (ePub)

Publisher: Health Communications, Inc.
      3201 S.W. 15th Street
      Deerfield Beach, FL 33442–8190

Cover photo © Olivia Brent
Cover design by Larissa Hise Henoch
Interior design and formatting by Lawna Patterson Oldfield

CONTENTS

INTRODUCTION

If you or someone you love is at risk for or has been diagnosed with breast cancer, rest assured that you have powerful healing medicine in the food you eat every day. The reality is that certain foods are nature's cancer-fighters because they are rich in cancer-healing phytochemicals (natural plant chemicals). Not only are they helpful in preventing cancer, but certain fruits, vegetables, seeds, herbs, and spices are rich in nutrients that are proven to inhibit cancer by actually turning off cancer genes and reducing cancer cell growth. These compounds can change the course of cancer.

In fact, many of the more progressive cancer clinics worldwide are starting to incorporate this research into their nutrition protocols to support and empower their patients throughout treatment. Targeting nutrition by prescribing nutrients based on an individual's needs not only supports healing but also enhances treatment efficacy.

As a clinical nutritionist specializing in medical nutrition therapy, I have been developing protocols and dietary guidelines for more than twenty years. Early in my career, it became clear to me that my cancer patients needed answers to their dietary quandaries. Many of them were unable to eat heated foods because the smells triggered nausea, so they frequently preferred cold foods. Some of my patients reported that they couldn't eat much at one sitting

1

so I made sure that the foods I recommended for them were nutrient dense, without extra carbohydrates and unnecessary bulk. Most of them were avoiding dairy products as they tend to increase mucus production and many of my new patients needed to gain muscle weight that had been lost due to treatment.

I could see that I would need to find creative ways to help them get proper nutrition. Some of the nutrient deficiencies that my patients were experiencing were very serious, such as cachexia, which is a wasting syndrome characterized by weight loss, muscle atrophy, fatigue, weakness, and loss of appetite. Cachexia not only affects quality of life but is also estimated to be the cause of death in 15 to 20 percent of all cancer patients. The treatment for this type of muscle loss is protein powder (amino acids) and specifically creatine, so I began adding protein powders to the smoothie formulas I created for them. Once I saw how quickly a targeted approach to nutrition could reverse a condition, I became focused on personalized medical nutrition therapy.

Most patients have nutrient deficiencies at the time of diagnosis. For example, large-scale studies have found that almost all women have vitamin D deficiency when they are first diagnosed with breast cancer. Vitamin D is needed for breast health as it plays key roles in immune function and breast tissue integrity. When our vitamin D levels drop below normal, we are in a carcinogenic state with a higher risk for developing breast cancer. By targeting and correcting deficiencies, we can dramatically change our health. This is true for specific nutrients and for broader nutrient categories, such as antioxidants and minerals.

A poor diet not only increases the risk for cancer but also reduces the ability to heal from cancer. The average American diet contains processed foods, chemicals, agricultural pesticides, and lots of sugar and hydrogenated fats, all of which are associated with cancer risk. This type of diet leads to inflammation, which is a leading underlying cause of cancer development and the most common cause of fatigue in cancer patients. My smoothie recipes are chock-full of antioxidants and phytochemicals that reduce inflammation. Both patients and readers who drink these smoothies daily report greater energy and less fatigue.

Creating functional smoothies containing active compounds has become a passion of mine, having seen the dramatic difference these drinks can make in an individual's health. Part of my process is to cull hundreds of studies on food nutrients found to affect recovery in various ways. First, I consider my patients' primary health concerns—for example, the side effects of chemo, which may include nausea, inflammation, fatigue, and muscle loss—and then I review the research to learn which food nutrients have been proven to support these conditions.

I pay attention to contraindicated foods that can wreak havoc for those with breast cancer. Some breast cancer subtypes require that the diet also be free of phytoestrogens, which are plant compounds that mimic hormones and stimulate the growth of cancer cells.

Since dairy products increase the growth of some types of breast cancer cells, I recommend cultured coconut milk, almond milk, or hemp milk instead of dairy. My recipes are void of processed sugar and unhealthy fats and are free of common allergenic foods, such as gluten, corn, dairy, and soy.

I also take into consideration the synergistic effects of nutrient compounds in the ingredients. Pairing food nutrients can actually amplify the healing power of your smoothies. For instance, black pepper increases the anti-inflammatory effects of turmeric by up to 2,000 percent and vitamin C enhances absorption of the mineral iron by sixfold. Therefore, combining iron-rich foods like Swiss chard, cashews, and bok choy with foods containing vitamin C, such as citrus and greens, will increase the health effects of iron. This is no small matter, as iron deficiency anemia is a common health problem in the United States and Canada.

A more exotic anti-inflammatory combination that has been used for thousands of years is turmeric with black pepper. Turmeric, the yellow spice used in curries, is rich in the phytochemical curcumin, which becomes more bioavailable when ingested along with piperine in black pepper. In addition, carnosic acid in rosemary enhances the effects of curcumin. Recent studies have also proven that the phytochemicals limonene and cineole, which are found in cardamom, enhance the effects of indole-3-carbinol (I3C), present in kale and other brassica family vegetables.

Prebiotics, which are the nondigestible fibers that feed probiotics, such as acidophilus and bifidophilus, support the growth of microbes in the gastro-intestinal tract. Most of the fruits and vegetables used in these recipes contain prebiotics, such as betaglucans from strawberries. This means that adding probiotics to plant-based smoothies will help activate those microbes in your body.

Having a healthy amount of microbes in the gut is necessary for proper digestion. An efficient digestive tract contains a wide variety of microbial strains that assist in digestion. Probiotics also enhance the effects of certain nutrients, for example, they metabolize anthocyanins from berries and pomegranate.

I find these nutrient and microbial interactions to be endlessly fascinating. A few decades ago, when I first started making smoothies, there was limited research available. Today there are studies being published daily from around the globe that direct our food nutrient choices for healing cancer. From these, I choose the studies that provide the most direct dietary guidance.

Some of these studies are done on animals, which is not only heartbreaking but also doesn't always provide information that is applicable to humans. Laboratory investigations with human cancer cells in petri dishes provide more direct proof of efficacy than many animal studies. Reports from human trials and correlational studies are the most revealing, as they involve direct testing of nutrients in humans, and they draw connections between nutrients and the health of populations.

Researchers are getting so specific in their recommendations that they often provide dose details in the conclusion of the study. This is the gold that I am digging for when I am slogging through hundreds of studies. When I come across a report that provides the exact amount of a specific food used in the study that led to a positive health outcome (reduction in cancer, in this case), I can then replicate that dosage in a smoothie. For example, one recent study found that just two to three stone fruits per day (e.g., apricots, peaches, and plums) reduced the growth of breast cancer in the study's participants.

I build my ingredients list from new research so that my recipes contain only effective cancer-supporting ingredients. I then use the USDA (United States Department of Agriculture) database to find the foods that contain the highest concentration of these desired food nutrients. To ensure that the ingredients I use are not contaminated with agricultural chemicals or depleted of nutrients through processing, I choose whole, unprocessed, organic, and non-GMO foods.

The final step to creating my "functional" smoothies is to take my ingredients to the kitchen, where I spend hundreds of hours developing recipes. And, voilà: the finished product is a variety of powerful, healthy recipes that target breast cancer.

Patients who drink my smoothies daily often report their mood and blood sugar levels are more stable and that they have more focus and motivation. They also report that their energy has increased enough that they are able to work and exercise throughout treatment.

If you want to take a proactive approach to preventing or healing cancer, one of the most effective steps you can take is to drink a breast cancer smoothie each day. It is my hope that you not only enjoy these recipes but that they fortify you to enjoy vibrant health.

CHAPTER 1

BREAST CANCER NUTRITION OVERVIEW

A breast cancer healing diet contains certain nutrients and avoids specific toxins and hormones. It is based on whole-plant foods and contains protein, minimizes sugar, and excludes synthetic compounds, such as chemical sweeteners, colorings, preservatives, or plastic residue from packaging.

The human body is in a constant state of change. Cells are dividing and growing and replacing older and damaged cells around the clock, so continually replacing nutritional components is critical. Food nutrients are crucial for healthy cell development. Most diets are deficient in breast cancer protective compounds. These smoothie recipes have concentrated amounts of the natural compounds needed to eliminate cancer cells and form a strong defense against new cancer cell development.

However, when significant nutrient deficiencies develop, or when nutrients are needed in therapeutic doses, supplementation may be required. When nutrient levels drop low enough, supplements may be needed for a short period of time to reverse the deficiency. But after supplementation, healthy nutrient levels can be maintained with food.

Keep in mind that these nutrients can only provide benefits if they are present in the body at the time of cell division, which is happening constantly. Therefore, it is important to add them to your daily diet by making them part of your routine. For example, you might want to make a smoothie first thing in the morning, or you may wish to have a smoothie each afternoon as a pick-me-up, or you may crave something sweet after a meal. A smoothie could become a treat you can savor while watching a movie or reading a book in the evening.

Deciding how many smoothies to drink each day depends on your diet and current nutrient status. Some nutrients are stored in the body while others are used quickly and the excess excreted. If you are working with a nutritionist or integrated care practitioner, they may perform lab tests to determine whether you are currently deficient in any specific areas. They will be able to use the results from your tests to guide you in increasing the intake of the compounds that your body currently needs.

If you eat a whole foods diet rich in high-protein plants you may only need to drink one smoothie per day. If you aren't sure whether you currently have vitamin, mineral, or amino acid deficiencies, start with two smoothies per day, for example, one in the morning and one in the late afternoon or evening. If you suspect that your diet is lacking, perhaps because you are unable to eat enough of the right foods, you may want to boost your intake by drinking three smoothies per day.

There is an increased need for nutrients during treatment and throughout the healing process. These include protein, fiber, minerals, vitamins, anti-oxidants, and essential fatty acids. Dietary protein is one of the three key macronutrients, along with carbohydrates and fats. Protein is made up of amino acids, which are needed for immune function, wound healing, and energy support. Stock your kitchen with high-protein plant foods to add to smoothies, as cancer increases the need for protein by up to 25 percent.

There are several protein foods that work well in smoothies. Chia seed and hulled hemp seed are rich in the omega-3 fatty acids that help reduce inflammation. This is important, because inflammation increases the risk for cancer and is a common cause of fatigue for cancer survivors. Protein supplements such as pea- and rice-based powders blend well and add a creamy base to smoothies. Choose vegan, low-sugar products when possible.

Keep sugar intake low as it increases breast cancer cell growth and metastasis. Avoid sweeteners, such as table sugar, maple syrup, agave, and honey. Keep in mind that synthetic sweeteners, such as aspartame and Splenda, should be avoided, as they are chemicals and linked to a host of health issues, including joint pain, headaches, diabetes, and microflora imbalance.

Nutrients play important roles in breast cancer prevention and treatment. They are cofactors in many biological processes throughout the body. Nutrient deficiencies not only cause malnutrition but reduce the efficacy of medications, hinder proper function of the endocrine and immune pathways, and increase the growth and spread of breast cancer cells.

Naturally occurring food nutrients, such as carotenoids, probiotics, and antioxidants, all play a role in healing breast cancer. Boost intake of these nutrients with greens, cantaloupe, stone fruit, cultured coconut milk, and wild blueberries. By making these simple ingredients part of your daily diet, you are ensuring that these nutrients are available as needed for your body's healing processes.

Most of the recipes are fruit-based because fruits contain proven nutrients for breast cancer. However, greens, beets, cucumbers, tomatoes, and other vegetables can be added to any smoothie. Vegetables are generally low in sugar and most contain minerals and antioxidants so they are a valuable addition to smoothies, even if they haven't yet been studied for their breast cancer benefits in a comprehensive way.

Fats are also an important nutrient addition to smoothies. Fats and proteins help reduce sugar cravings and stabilize blood sugar levels. Sources of essential fatty acids (EFAs) that are supportive for breast health include primrose oil, borage oil, algae oil, and hemp and chia seeds.

Choosing organic produce can be important, as many pesticides and herbicides are also highly toxic to breast tissue. Some crops, such as strawberries, are more heavily sprayed than others, so it is especially important to buy organic strawberries. For a list of the foods most heavily contaminated, as well as a list of produce that is sprayed the least, see *EWG.org* and the list on page 34.

Dairy is contraindicated for most types of breast cancer. Dairy foods, such as milk, ice cream, and whey protein powder, have been found to increase insulin-like growth factor (IGF-1) levels, which is linked to breast cancer cell growth. Also, milk and other dairy products have varying levels of naturally occurring estrogens that have the potential to mimic human hormones.

The cancer risk from dairy may be increased by genetically engineered bovine growth hormone (BGH), which is injected into most dairy cows to increase milk production. Organic dairy products may be safer because they are free of synthetic BGH and are currently being evaluated for their estrogenic effects on breast cancer patients. However, until there is more evidence, avoid dairy products altogether.

Plastic water bottles, plastic food packaging, and plastic food storage containers need to be avoided, as phthalates from plastic mimic estrogen, and some have the ability to stimulate breast cancer cells. Phthalates, such as bisphenol A (BPA), diethyl phthalates (DEP), and dibutyl phthalate (DBP), have been implicated in scientific studies as causative factors in breast cancer development and growth. Avoid plastic food containers, opting instead for stainless steel, glass, waxed paper, and cardboard containers.

Personalized Smoothies

Breast cancer develops because of multiple imbalances, which generally include genetics and environmental factors. You can personalize your smoothies to meet your individual needs based on your specific type of breast cancer.

Research shows that although all women need consistent intake of antioxidants, these nutrients are even more helpful for those who are premenopausal, as antioxidants reduce estrogen's effects on breast cancer cells. Most cases of premenopausal breast cancer are estrogen receptor positive (ER+). In fact, two-thirds of all breast cancer cases are ER+, so typical treatment strategies include estrogen reduction. Some foods provide bioactive compounds that support estrogen suppression. For example, kale is a food that helps bind with hormones and reduces estrogenic activity.

Many food nutrients have been proven to affect breast cancer cells by reducing their numbers, inhibiting their growth, and helping eradicate them from the body. Not only are the effects of food nutrients being studied to determine how they affect breast cancer but also their effects on specific subgroups. Nutrients are being used therapeutically for ER+, ER-, and TNBC (triple-negative breast cancer) subtypes, for example. Just as certain therapies can target certain types of cancer, smoothies can be customized by adding more of the nutrients known to help with your specific type of breast cancer. By enhancing your smoothies with the most effective nutrients for your condition, you can create a more powerful medicinal impact.

All of the foods listed below are rich in nutrients that are healthful for everyone, and none of these foods are harmful in any way, so don't feel you must strictly choose foods from your subtype list. The following is intended to inform you about the latest research because food nutrients are now proven to be effective therapeutically (as treatment). This becomes even more important when your doctor offers few treatment options. For example, TNBC is a hard-to-treat subtype with few pharmaceutical options.

Creating a personalized smoothie is easy. Start with one cup of your favorite liquid, such as green tea, currant juice, or coconut water; add one-half cup of fruit; one-half cup of greens; and a teaspoon of herbs/spices as recommended for your subtype to follow. If you are drinking smoothies for prevention, choose from any food category. A personalized smoothie each day can make a significant and immediate difference in your health.

You may even want to keep a diet diary and track your symptoms to help you identify just how much better you feel as you have your daily smoothies. You can do this by jotting down your symptoms, such as fatigue, weight gain, headaches, muscle pain, and dry mouth, then rate their severity on a scale of one to ten. It is easy to forget how bad we felt once we feel better.

Drink one to three of your own smoothies each day based on the following list and keep track of your symptoms for a few weeks. Then you can clearly see the difference these drinks can make in your overall health.

ER+ *(estrogen receptor positive)*

Antioxidant tannins and flavonoids (pomegranate seeds)
Antioxidants (berries and greens)
Ellagic acid (berries, peaches, grapes, and strawberries)
Isatin (plums and prunes)
Norathyriol (mango and mango skin)
Prebiotics (strawberries and garlic)
Probiotics (cultured coconut milk and cultured almond milk)
Quercetin (apples, including the skin)

PR+ *(progesterone receptor positive)*

Antioxidants (berries and greens)
Avoid dairy

ER- *(estrogen receptor negative)*

Carnosic acid (rosemary)

Curcumin (turmeric)

Antioxidants (greens, berries, and stone fruit)

HER2 (human epidermal growth factor receptor 2)

Indole-3-carbinol (kale)

TNBC (triple-negative breast cancer)

Naringin (citrus)

Hesperidin (citrus)

Antioxidants (blueberries)

BRCA1 and BRCA2 (breast cancer genes 1 and 2)

Antioxidants (greens, berries, and stone fruit)

Anti-inflammatory foods (rosemary, basil, citrus, berries, greens)

Avoid alcohol

Avoid sugar and other inflammatory foods

Avoid plastics (BPA)

Although this may feel like a lot to consider, it is worth the effort. Making these small, incremental changes to your diet can make a profound difference in recovery and long-term remission. Start with something simple, such as replacing your dairy milk with almond milk or stocking your freezer with blueberries so that you can easily add them to your daily smoothies. Even small dietary changes enhance healing, slow the development of cancer, increase energy, and help prevent recurrence.

Breast Cancer Healing Smoothie Recipes

Creating nutrient-dense smoothies requires a little planning. I've organized the recipes by food type to minimize the number of ingredients needed to make smoothies for several days in a row.

Frozen ingredients are convenient because they have such a long shelf life and can be kept at the ready for months. Fresh ingredients require more frequent trips to the store. You may need to shop for fresh ingredients twice a week but frozen ingredients only once a month.

The most important breast cancer food nutrient categories include antioxidants, specifically carotenoids and polyphenols. These nutrients are concentrated in specific plant foods, including stone fruit, citrus, and berries, so many of the recipes focus on these nutrient powerhouses.

Each recipe contains a description of the drink's flavors to help you identify smoothies to fit your taste. The ingredients are listed in order of the largest quantity first, such as fruit or liquid, down to the tiniest quantity, such as spices. Smoothie ingredients can be added in any order unless your blender motor isn't strong enough to grind through dry, fibrous, or frozen ingredients. In this case, it is best to add the liquid first to reduce pressure on the blender blades. With a little preparation, you can blend drinks in minutes. Consider making tea cubes and freezing your produce, such as bananas, when possible.

Each recipe has been created to combine the most nutritious ingredients that deliver protein, fiber, nutrients, and rich flavor without much sugar.

Recipes are intended as guides. Try the recipes and then alter them to meet your needs by adding more spices, protein, or greens, for example. Add more liquid if the flavor is too intense and opt for fresh rather than frozen ingredients if you prefer.

The fruits included in these recipes have been chosen for their nutrients, which provide direct action against breast cancer cells. This way we avoid using any filler ingredients merely for flavor. All of the ingredients add a medicinal punch against breast cancer cells. Every sip is a rich concoction of nutrients that enters the bloodstream via the stomach and intestines. Once the nutrients reach the bloodstream, they are delivered to cells throughout the body, sending signals to your genes, which then send instructions to your cells. I've chosen nutrients that start the chain of command to turn off cancer cell division and growth. This is called epigenetic action.

These fruit nutrients are critical and cannot be obtained from vegetables, so inclusion of fruit is very important in a breast cancer diet. However, fruits contain various amounts of sugar, which is why they're so sweet and delicious. The challenge is to include fruits that deliver the most potent, cancer-fighting nutrients while containing the lowest amount of sugar possible.

One recent, thrilling nutrient discovery is that fruit peels, such as banana, citrus, and mango skin, contain concentrated amounts of the same nutrients that are found in the pulp and juice. If you use organic fruit, which is free of pesticide residue, you can blend the fruit skin into your smoothie, which not only boosts nutrient levels but also fiber.

When we blend whole fruits and vegetables, the fiber is blended into the smoothie. This is in contrast to juicing, which separates the fiber from the juice. The advantage of ingesting the fiber is that the soluble and insoluble fiber slows the absorption of the plants' natural sugars into the blood.

The concern about ingesting too much sugar too quickly is that a load of sugar can cause a blood sugar spike. We want to avoid high blood sugar because it is damaging to our blood vessels and triggers inflammation, a driver of cancer cells.

When we eat whole fruits, we are ingesting the fruit sugar in a matrix of fiber, which changes how we absorb the sugar. Herein lies the magic of fiber from whole foods. Fiber slows the release of the sugar so that our bodies have time to use it for important biological activities, including fueling brain and muscle cells. Thus, high-fiber foods are the perfect delivery vehicle for our main source of energy, which is sugar.

The issue of slow absorption of food sugars is important, especially for those with diabetes, hypoglycemia, and cancer. Therefore, nutritionists have been working on ways to determine how much the foods we eat will affect blood sugar levels. Several systems have been developed over the years that are still in use today: (a) the glycemic index, which rates foods from the most sugary to the least, and (b) the more sophisticated glycemic load, which estimates how much a food will raise a person's blood glucose level based on sugar and fiber content. More recently, the term "net carbs" is being used to determine the amount of carbs that produce sugar, rather than carbs from fiber, in a particular food or combination of foods. This is a simple calculation of taking the total number of grams of carbohydrates and subtracting the number of grams of fiber to get the total number of grams of carbohydrates.

Net carbs have been provided in the nutrition facts information given with each recipe so that the total number of actual carbs can be seen easily. While fiber technically counts as carbohydrates, it is considered a "nonimpact" carbohydrate, the type that doesn't raise blood sugar levels. Fiber not only doesn't contribute to an increase of sugar in the blood, it also reduces the risk for blood sugar spikes, as it slows the absorption of other carbohydrates from the digestive tract. Therefore, net carbs values are a more accurate reflection of the actual "impact carbs" in a food or recipe. The recipes in this book all have a net carb value of twenty or less.

Note that the nutrition analysis reflects the number of servings in the recipe. Of course, recipes for one can be doubled and those for two can be cut in half. The nutrition facts provided with each recipe were produced by careful analysis with Food Processor Nutrition Analysis Software by ESHA Research for accuracy.

All of the ingredients used in my recipes have been well researched and provide proven benefits. The amount of the ingredients used in each recipe has been determined, in most cases, by the dose used to produce results in laboratory studies and in human subjects in trials. Keep in mind that food nutrients support healing when cells are exposed to them consistently. Think of your daily smoothie as a nutrient infusion. These nutrients can change body chemistry, creating an internal environment that no longer supports breast cancer growth.

Targeted nutrition not only enhances healing by inhibiting cancer cell development and growth but also produces noticeable effects, such as better digestion, improved sleep, and more energy.

You can change the course of your cancer by starting your daily smoothie routine today!

How to Use This Book

As you're reading, you may have questions about the definition of a term, the research behind a recommendation, or about alternative ingredients. There is a Glossary of Terms in the back of the book and a research reference section that is organized by food type. This makes it easy to find the studies on a specific food.

Also, Chapter 4, Ingredients: Purchasing, Prepping, and Storing, provides a more involved list of foods that contain healing or preventative nutrients. Refer to the list for information about where to find these foods and how to prepare and store them.

Chapter 5, The Recipes, is broken into eleven sets of smoothies, each focusing on a base ingredient, such as apricot nectar or green tea. If you work your way through the recipes in order, you'll be buying ingredients for several smoothies at a time. For example, the first set of recipes is centered around apples and apple juice, the second set is on apricot nectar, and so on. This means less trips to the store and less wasted food.

An explanation of the health benefits of the ingredients accompanies each recipe. This is where you'll find tips about food nutrients and how they act in

various ways to prevent and inhibit the process of breast cancer. Tips throughout the book explain how food nutrients increase an immune response to
breast cancer cells, reduce blood flow to cancer tissues, turn off genetic signaling pathways, and cause apoptosis, which is literally the destruction of
existing cancer cells.

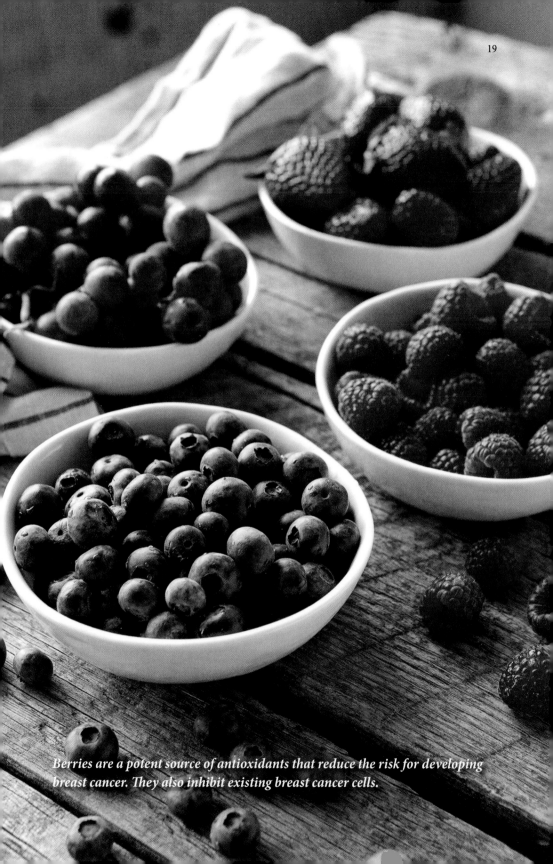

Berries are a potent source of antioxidants that reduce the risk for developing breast cancer. They also inhibit existing breast cancer cells.

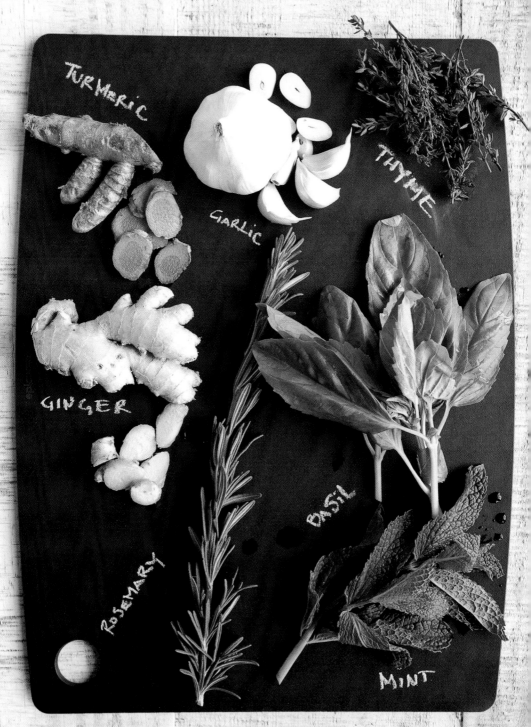

Herbs are potent sources of anticancer compounds.

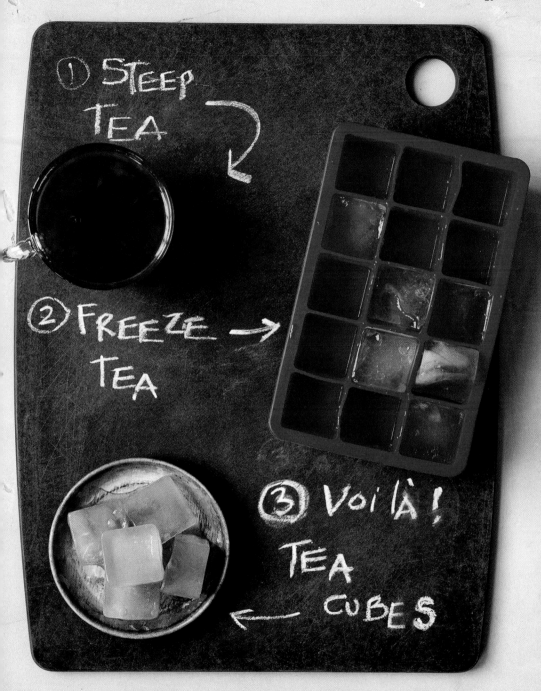

Green tea can be frozen into cubes and stored in the freezer for a handy addition of antioxidants for smoothies (see page 36 for details).

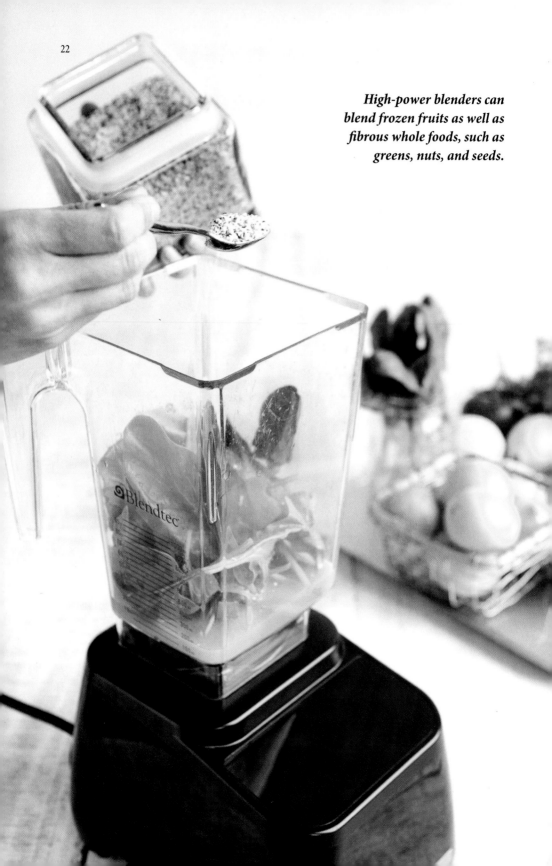

High-power blenders can blend frozen fruits as well as fibrous whole foods, such as greens, nuts, and seeds.

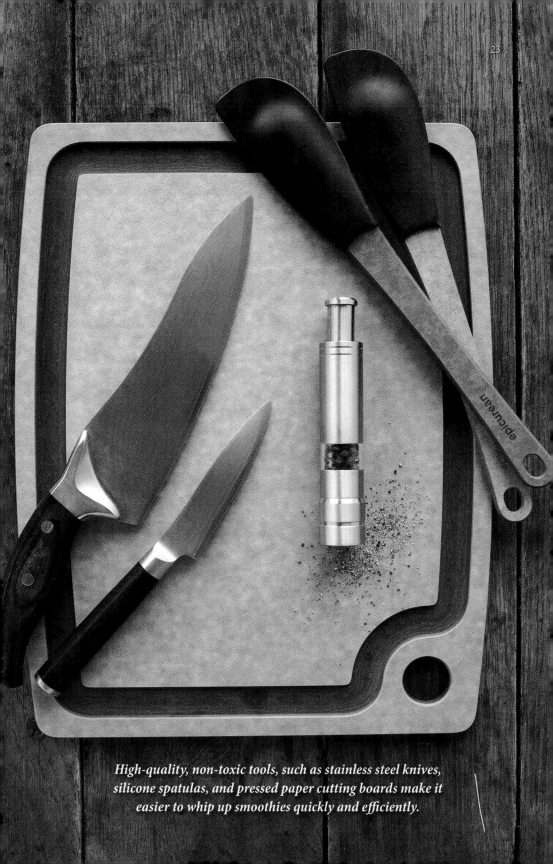

High-quality, non-toxic tools, such as stainless steel knives, silicone spatulas, and pressed paper cutting boards make it easier to whip up smoothies quickly and efficiently.

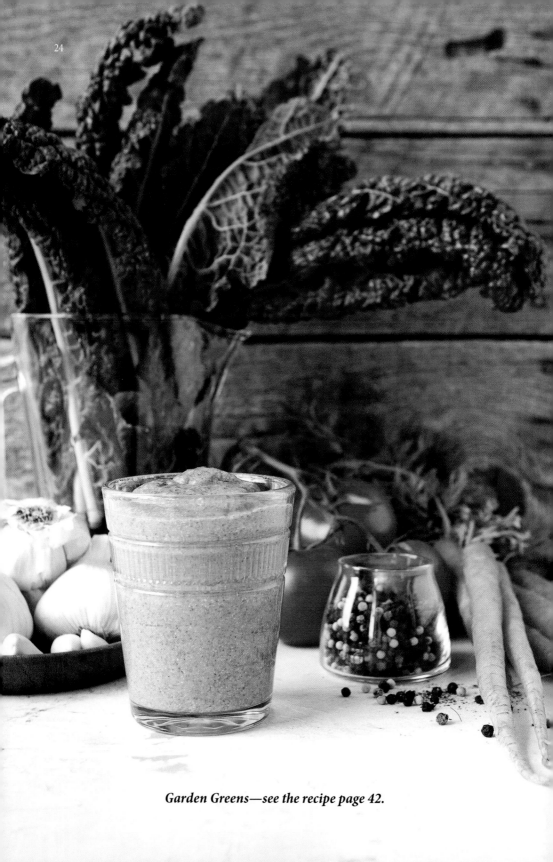

Garden Greens—see the recipe page 42.

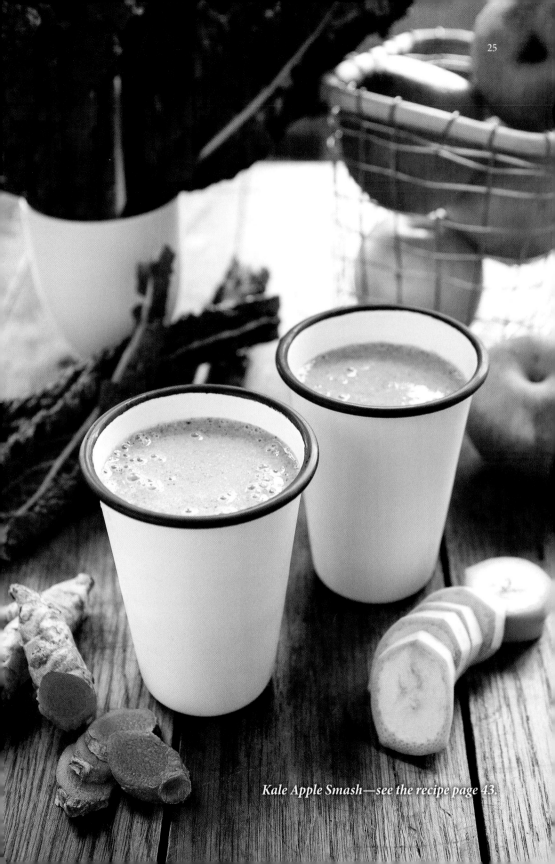

Kale Apple Smash—see the recipe page 43.

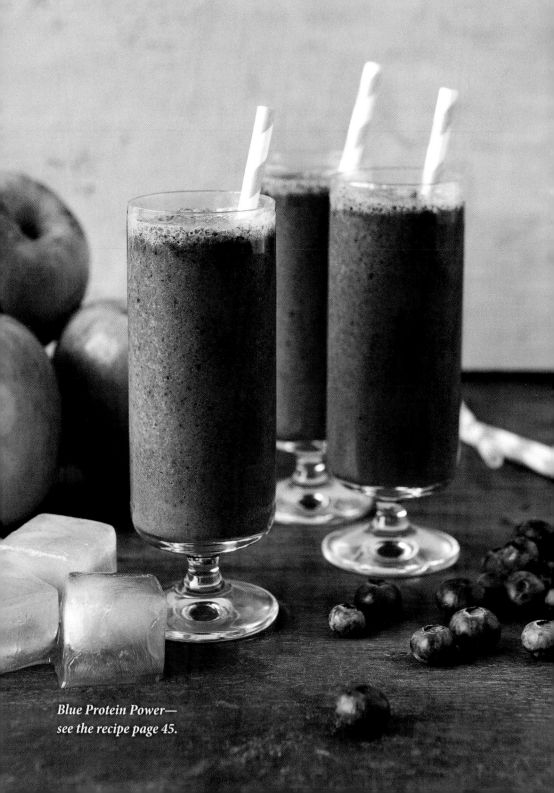

Blue Protein Power—
see the recipe page 45.

CHAPTER 2

THE HEALTHY KITCHEN

The basic equipment needed for making smoothies is a blender, a sharp knife, and a nontoxic cutting board. Besides those key tools, you may also want to have a spatula for scraping down the sides of the blender, a few ice trays for making iced tea cubes, waxed paper bags for storing fruits in the freezer, and measuring cups and spoons. Use glass, not plastic cups, for serving your drinks. There are many gorgeous, nontoxic tools these days, that make it easier than ever to set up a clean kitchen for smoothie making.

The most important smoothie kitchen tool is, of course, the blender. High-power or high-performance blenders feature incredibly powerful motors—700 watts—or more. Vitamix and Blendtec are two popular high-power blenders. Small blenders can be powerful too. For example, the TriBest blender has a small base and uses Mason jars as the pitcher. If the pitcher breaks, you can use any Mason jar with their adapters as a replacement. I love the idea of dual-use kitchen tools, as this saves space in the cupboards. It's also more affordable than the bigger blenders and tiny enough to fit in any kitchen cupboard.

Even though some of these high-power blenders have a heat function, I don't recommend using heat with a plastic pitcher because heat increases the leaching of toxins from plastic, which allows these particles to migrate into the food. Avoid plastics when possible by opting for a blender with a glass pitcher.

If you already have a blender with a plastic pitcher, use it for cold foods only. For example, avoid pouring hot tea directly into a plastic blender pitcher. Instead, brew the tea and let it cool. Then pour the room temperature tea into the blender pitcher, or it can be poured into silicone ice cube trays and frozen for later use. If your current blender has a plastic pitcher, you may be able to replace the plastic pitcher with a large Mason glass jar, as they fit most blenders.

Handheld blenders are small, so they can be stored in a drawer and are easy to clean. They work well when making a smoothie for one person. Just combine your ingredients in a bowl or a tall stainless steel cup and blend. They can be rinsed in seconds. Most of the kitchen tool manufacturers, including Cuisinart, Hamilton Beach, and Proctor-Silex offer hand blenders.

Buying nontoxic kitchen tools is important, as heavy metals and plastics can cause breast cancer cells to grow and spread. Always be sure to use nontoxic measuring tools, as other types can be sources of breast cancer toxins. Avoid aluminum and metal-plated measuring cups and spoons. Aluminum becomes a toxin when it builds up in body tissues, and it appears to have an affinity for breast tissue. This means that it accumulates in breasts, where it can cause physiologic harm. About half of those with breast cancer have a genetic weakness that makes them even more susceptible to the accumulation of heavy metals, such as aluminum.

Glass or stainless steel measuring cups and spoons are nontoxic alternatives to the aluminum and plastic varieties. Avoid the other types of metal tools as they often deteriorate over time, allowing flakes of metallic material to contaminate food with toxic metals.

Spatulas can be helpful for scraping those last delicious spoonfuls of a smoothie from a blender pitcher. Just be sure to avoid plastic spatulas and instead opt for high-heat resistant silicone spatulas, which are nontoxic, heat resistant up to 500°F/260°C, and dishwasher safe.

A large cutting board allows enough room to safely prepare produce. However, cutting boards are often made from toxic plastics that develop abrasions with use and release bits of plastic into food. Although wood is natural, it isn't the best option, as it often harbors potentially dangerous bacteria that can grow in the wet wood fiber. A healthier option is pressed-paper cutting boards. They last for years and won't dull knives as quickly as harder cutting-board materials. Keep two different cutting boards if you prepare meat in your home. Keep one board solely for meat and another for produce, such as fresh herbs, vegetables, and fruit. If possible, run cutting boards through the dishwasher after each use to sterilize them.

A high-quality knife allows you to chop and prep produce quickly without a lot of mess or frustration. Some prefer a small paring knife, but I use an eight-inch chef's knife for almost all of my chopping and slicing. Hand washing your knife will help it stay sharp longer than if you clean it in the dishwasher. Shun, Messermeister, and Wüsthof make quality knives.

Store ingredients in nontoxic, airtight containers. Dry foods, such as nuts and oatmeal, can be stored in BPA-free plastic containers, but wet foods leach toxins from plastics, so they should be stored in glass containers. High-quality glass storage containers, such as the old standby, Duralex, are shock resistant and can go from freezer to microwave without breaking. This is helpful if you have stored produce in the freezer and need to thaw it in the microwave before blending. Waxed paper bags or BPA-free food storage bags can be used for freezer items rather than plastic food storage bags.

If possible, install a water filter, preferably a solid carbon filtration system, at your tap to remove chlorine, heavy metals, and other environmental contaminants from your drinking water and ice cubes.

CHAPTER 3

SMOOTHIE-MAKING STEPS

A successful smoothie can be made in just a few basic steps. Once you have mastered the basics, you may want to purchase a few quality tools to simplify the process and reduce frustration, such as a chef's knife and a large pressed-paper cutting board.

No. 1: Shop

Review the recipes you'll be making for the week. Scan through the recipes and check your refrigerator, freezer, and fruit bowl to see which ingredients you already have on hand and which you'll need to put on your grocery list. If you have trouble identifying or locating an unusual food, look it up under Ingredients: Purchasing, Prepping, and Storing in Chapter 4, which may provide more clues.

No. 2: Prep

After shopping for your ingredients, prepare your produce by removing the organic stickers and pits (if necessary), washing greens, chopping vegetables and herbs, and making the iced tea cubes and other items that need to be done ahead of time. The Ingredients section in Chapter 4 also provides purchasing, preparation, and storage details for each ingredient.

No. 3: Combine

When you're ready to make your smoothie, place your ingredients, such as fruits, vegetables, liquids, seeds, protein powder, and other dry ingredients in a blender or food processor. If you have a high-power blender, you can add everything at once without much thought. If you have a lower-power blender, you can reduce stress on the motor by adding liquids first, thawing frozen fruits for a few minutes before blending, and resting the motor if you can tell it is struggling. Also, adding more liquid as you blend will soften the ingredients.

The recipes in this book were made with high-power Blendtec and Vitamix blenders. They require less liquid to macerate tougher foods, such as whole fruits, nuts, and frozen produce. Blenders with duller blades or less power may require slight alterations to the recipes. For example, if your blender has a hard time with whole apples, you may want to peel and core them first. If frozen fruit bogs down your blender, just add more liquid or use raw fruit rather than frozen.

No. 4: Blend

Blend your ingredients to your desired consistency.

No. 5: Clean

Rinse the blender pitcher and put it away or run it through the dishwasher to sterilize it.

CHAPTER 4

INGREDIENTS: PURCHASING, PREPPING, AND STORING

Use this section as a reference for identifying some of the less famil-iar items and for help with purchasing, preparing, and storing each ingredient.

The Organic Option

Fruits and vegetables may be heavily sprayed with herbicides and pes-ticides. Some fruits, such as apples and strawberries, are the most heavily sprayed, while others, such as avocado and grapefruit, require minimal chemicals in their growing process. The Environmental Working Group (EWG) provides an up-to-date "Clean Fifteen" list of the least sprayed pro-duce and a "Dirty Dozen" list of the most heavily sprayed produce on their website at *EWG.org* (see the lists below). Use these lists to help you decide which produce should be purchased with the organic label, which assures that no agricultural chemicals were used on them.

Dirty Dozen: EWG's Shopper's Guide to Pesticides in Produce

1. Strawberries
2. Apples
3. Nectarines
4. Peaches
5. Celery
6. Grapes
7. Cherries
8. Spinach
9. Tomatoes
10. Bell Peppers
11. Cherry Tomatoes
12. Cucumbers

Clean Fifteen: EWG's Shopper's Guide to Pesticides in Produce

1. Avocados
2. Corn
3. Pineapples
4. Cabbage
5. Sweet Peas
6. Onions
7. Asparagus
8. Mangoes
9. Papayas
10. Kiwi
11. Eggplant
12. Honeydew
13. Grapefruit
14. Cantaloupe
15. Cauliflower

Whole Foods Without Additives

Look for juice labels that state 100% juice with no sugar, preservatives, or synthetic sweeteners. Buy juices in glass rather than plastic. It is also possible to make your own juice at home with a juicer, such as Novis Vita Juicer, using whole fruits and vegetables.

Washing Produce

It's wise to rinse all produce well for at least thirty seconds to remove bacteria and fungus before chopping or adding it to a smoothie. Some produce, such as melons, carry more risk than other fruits, and can be vectors for salmonella if not washed properly. It is prudent to scrub the outside skin of fruit and rinse the cut pieces well, which helps flush away pathogenic organisms that may have been pulled into the fruit by the knife. This is especially important for those who are immune-compromised and vulnerable to infections from a burdened immune system, such as those with cancer and/ or who are undergoing cancer treatment.

Leafy greens such as kale should be washed well under running water and wrapped wet in a clean cloth towel, which will help them stay fresh in the refrigerator's crisper drawer for several days.

Storage of Liquids

If you've opened a container of liquid, such as coconut water, and are not able to use it up within a few days, you can keep the remainder from spoiling by freezing it. Pour the liquid into ice cube trays, and once frozen, you can pop out the cubes into waxed paper or BPA-free food storage bags, where they will stay fresh in the freezer for months. This trick works equally well for brewed green tea and fruit juices.

Freezing Produce

Frozen fruit prepped specifically for smoothies, such as pitted cherries and peaches, are available in bags in the freezer section of the store. If you have a surplus of fresh-picked or store-bought fresh produce that you can't eat before it becomes overripe, you can freeze it. Prepare the fruit by removing the pit, seeds, or rind. When freezing berries, rinse them well and let them dry for at least one hour on a clean cloth towel so they are dry when frozen, which keeps them from clumping.

Smoothie Cubes

Make smoothies ahead of time and pour them into ice trays. Pop out cubes and drop them into the blender with a liquid, such as green tea, juice, or water, and blend for a quick smoothie when you're short on time. You may want to prep this way for yourself when you have treatments planned or if you just don't have the energy to spend time in the kitchen. By doing a little prep work ahead of time, you can stay on your smoothie program during days when you're tired or busy.

CHAPTER 5

THE RECIPES

APPLE SMOOTHIES

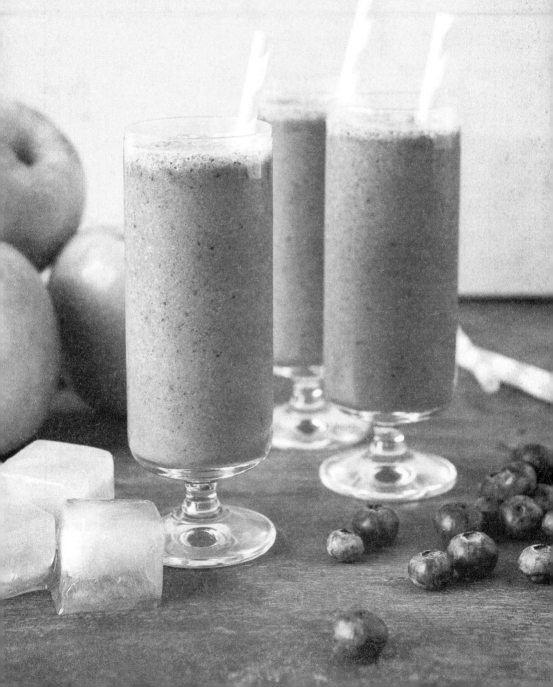

APPLE RASPBERRY TEA

*T*his slightly sweet smoothie is well balanced, with apple and berry flavors and sophisticated tannic tea undertones.

Quercetin, found abundantly in apples, promotes apoptosis of breast cancer cells and is protective against tumor growth.

SERVES ❷

½ apple

½ cup unfiltered apple juice

½ cup black raspberries

½ cup green tea ice cubes

2 tablespoons hulled hemp seed

2 teaspoons lemon juice

¼ teaspoon turmeric powder

Combine all ingredients in a high-power blender or food processor and blend until smooth. Drink immediately.

Nutrition Facts *(per serving)*

Calories 140; Fat 5; Protein 4; Carbs 21; Fiber 5; Net Carbs 16

Research Study

P. Bulzomi, A. Bolli, P. Galluzzo, et al. (2012). The naringenin-induced proapoptotic effect in breast cancer cell lines holds out against a high bisphenol a background. *Journal of Nutrition* 64 (8): 690–96.

QUERCETIN QUENCHER

This cool combination tastes like fresh apples with layers of summer fruit flavor.

Quercetin, found in apples, can modulate estrogen receptor activities and promotes apoptosis of breast cancer cells.

SERVES **2**

½ apple

½ cup unfiltered apple juice

½ cup frozen cherries

½ cup frozen peaches

2 tablespoons chia seed

¼ teaspoon turmeric powder

Combine all ingredients in a high-power blender or food processor and blend until smooth. Drink immediately.

Nutrition Facts *(per serving)*

Calories 150; Fat 5; Protein 4; Carbs 26; Fiber 8; Net Carbs 18

Research Study

C. Huang, S. Y. Lee, C. L. Lin, et al. (2013). Co-treatment with quercetin and 1,2,3,4,6-penta-O-galloyl-β-D-glucose causes cell cycle arrest and apoptosis in human breast cancer MDA- MB-231 and AU565 cells. *Journal of Agricultural and Food Chemistry* 61 (26): 6430–45.

GARDEN GREENS

*T*his garden combination has a creamy base and a little nutty flavor from
the sunflower seeds and hemp. See photo page 24.

Sunflower seeds are a
rich source of protein and
beneficial plant lignans
that appear to suppress
the growth of breast
cancer cells by reducing
the tumor-stimulating
effects of circulating
estrogen.

SERVES ❷

½ cup unfiltered apple juice

½ cup tomatoes

½ cup greens

½ cup green tea ice cubes

2 tablespoons sunflower seed

2 tablespoons hulled hemp seed

Combine all ingredients in a high-
power blender or food processor and
blend until smooth. Drink immediately.

Nutrition Facts *(per serving)*

Calories 140; Fat 7; Protein 6; Carbs 12; Fiber 2; Net Carbs 10

Research Study

R. Suzuki, T. Rylander-Rudqvist, S. Saji, et al. (2008). Dietary lignans and postmenopausal breast cancer risk by estrogen receptor
status: A prospective cohort study of Swedish women. *British Journal of Cancer* 98 (3): 636–40.

KALE APPLE SMASH

*F*rosty, creamy, and sweet, this smoothie has a delicious, fresh garden greens flavor and a bright green color. See photo page 25.

Indole-3-carbinol (I3C) and diindolylmethane (DIM) are phytochemicals found in kale. They have demonstrated exceptional anticancer effects against hormone-sensitive breast cancer cells. Additionally, phytochemicals in cardamom have been found to increase the bioavailability of I3C and DIM when eaten with kale.

SERVES **1**

½ frozen banana

½ cup unfiltered apple juice

½ cup kale

½ cup green tea ice cubes

2 tablespoons hulled hemp seed

1 teaspoon lemon juice

¼ teaspoon cardamom powder

Combine all ingredients in a high-power blender or food processor and blend until smooth. Drink immediately.

Nutrition Facts *(per serving)*

Calories 140; Fat 5; Protein 4; Carbs 22; Fiber 2; Net Carbs 20

Research Study

A. Acharya, I. Das, S. Singh, et al. (2010). Chemopreventive properties of indole-3-carbinol, diindolylmethane and other constituents of cardamom against carcinogenesis. *Recent Patents of Food, Nutrition and Agriculture* 2 (2): 166–77.

GOLDEN BANANA AND GREENS

*H*eady and lightly sweet, this green smoothie has the perfect balance of fruit and greens.

Women with higher circulating blood levels of alpha-carotene, beta-carotene, lutein, zeaxanthin, lycopene, and total carotenoids may have a reduced risk of breast cancer.

SERVES ❷

1 cup greens

½ frozen banana

½ cup unfiltered apple juice

¼ cup hulled hemp seed

¼ teaspoon turmeric powder

Combine all ingredients in a high-power blender or food processor and blend until smooth. Drink immediately.

Nutrition Facts *(per serving)*

Calories 200; Fat 9; Protein 8; Carbs 23; Fiber 3; Net Carbs 20

Research Study

A. H. Eliassen, S. J. Hendrickson, L. A. Brinton, et al. (2012). Circulating carotenoids and risk of breast cancer: Pooled analysis of eight prospective studies. *Journal of the National Cancer Institute* 104 (24): 1905–16.

BLUE PROTEIN POWER

*L*ightly sweet and creamy, this blue smoothie is rich in protein and fresh blueberry flavor and color (see photo page 26).

During the healing process from cancer, there is an increased need for protein intake. This recipe has a double hit of protein from the hemp and the protein powder. Apples and citrus fruits contain pectic oligosaccharides (POS) that inhibit breast cancer cell growth and trigger apoptosis in human breast cancer cells.

SERVES ❷

1 cup blueberries

½ cup green tea ice cubes

½ cup unfiltered apple juice

2 tablespoons hulled hemp seed

2 tablespoons protein powder

Combine all ingredients in a high-power blender or food processor and blend until smooth. Drink immediately.

Nutrition Facts *(per serving)*

Calories 180; Fat 6; Protein 11; Carbs 23; Fiber 6; Net Carbs 17

Research Study

L. Delphi, H. Sepehri, M. R. Khorramizadeh, et al. (2015). Pectic-oligosaccharides from apples induce apoptosis and cell cycle arrest in MDA-MB-231 cells, a model of human breast cancer. *Asian Pacific Organization for Cancer Prevention* 16 (13): 5265–71.

LEMON ROSEMARY TEA

*T*his light and lemony smoothie is slightly sweet with an herbal fragrance.

Green tea catechins suppress the growth of breast tumors.

SERVES ❷

1 cup green tea ice cubes

1 cup unfiltered apple juice

¼ cup hulled hemp seed

1 tablespoon lemon juice

1 teaspoon rosemary leaf powder

Combine all ingredients in a high-power blender or food processor and blend until smooth. Drink immediately.

Nutrition Facts *(per serving)*

Calories 90; Fat 5; Protein 4; Carbs 8; Fiber 1; Net Carbs 7

Research Study

E. C. Yiannakopoulou. (2013). Green tea catechins: Proposed mechanisms of action in breast cancer focusing on the interplay between survival and apoptosis. *Anticancer Agents Medicinal Chemistry* 14 (2): 290–95.

APRICOT
SMOOTHIES

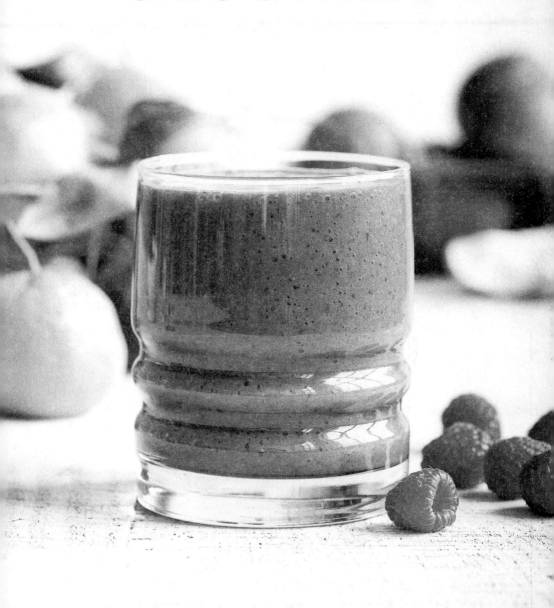

APRICOT GREEN TEA

*I*n this light and fresh smoothie, the subtle apple and green tea flavors
mingle with just a touch of citrus.

Apples contain quercetin
and triterpenoids that
reduce inflammation,
improve immune
response, and reduce
breast cancer cell growth.
These nutrients are found
in fresh apples, apple
skins, apple extracts, and
apple pulp.

Apricots and kale are rich
in breast cancer-protective
carotenoids.

SERVES ❷

½ apple

½ cup apricot nectar

½ cup kale

1 cup green tea ice cubes

2 tablespoons chia seed

1 teaspoon lemon juice

Combine all ingredients in a high-
power blender or food processor and
blend until smooth. Drink immediately.

Nutrition Facts *(per serving)*

Calories 130; Fat 5; Protein 4; Carbs 21; Fiber 7; Net Carbs 14

Research Studies

X. He, Y. Wang, H. Hu, et al. (2012). In vitro and in vivo antimammary tumor activities and mechanisms of the apple total triterpenoids. *Journal of Agricultural and Food Chemistry* 60 (37): 9430–36.

G. C. Kabat, M. Kim, L. L. Adams-Campbell, et al. (2009). Longitudinal study of serum carotenoid, retinol, and tocopherol concentrations in relation to breast cancer risk among postmenopausal women. *American Journal of Clinical Nutrition* 90 (1): 162–69.

TART APRICOT

*T*his smoothie has fresh apricot and banana flavors with a little golden turmeric and a light lemon finish.

Apple skins contain potent antiproliferative compounds that reduce human breast cancer cells by lowering inflammation and improving immune response. When researchers used apple peel extracts on cancer cells in the laboratory, they found that treatment resulted in a marked increase in maspin, a tumor suppressor protein that reduces cell invasion, metastasis, and angiogenesis. Spinach and apricot nectar also contain carotenoids that suppress breast cancer development.

SERVES ❷

1 apple

1 cup green tea ice cubes

½ cup apricot nectar

½ cup spinach

2 tablespoons chia seed

1 tablespoon lemon juice

½ teaspoon turmeric powder

Pinch of fresh ground black pepper

Combine all ingredients in a high-power blender or food processor and blend until smooth. Drink immediately.

Nutrition Facts *(per serving)*

Calories 140; Fat 5; Protein 4; Carbs 24; Fiber 8; Net Carbs 16

Research Study

S. Reagan-Shaw, D. Eggert, H. Mukhtar, et al. (2010). Antiproliferative effects of apple peel extract against cancer cells. *Nutrition and Cancer* 62 (4): 517–24.

WILD BLUEBERRY APRICOT

*T*his sweet, aromatic combination has deep blueberry and fruit flavors with a hint of spice. Perfection!

Apricots are a rich source of lycopene, an antioxidant carotenoid, which shows an array of biological effects, including anti-inflammatory, antimutagenic, and anticarcinogenic activities.

SERVES ❷

1 cup green tea ice cubes

½ cup apricot nectar

½ cup frozen wild blueberries

2 tablespoons hulled hemp seed

½ teaspoon turmeric powder

Pinch of fresh ground black pepper

Combine all ingredients in a high-power blender or food processor and blend until smooth. Drink immediately.

Nutrition Facts *(per serving)*

Calories 110; Fat 6; Protein 4; Carbs 13; Fiber 3; Net Carbs 10

Research Study

B. Yan, M. S. Lu, L. Wang, et al. (2016). Specific serum carotenoids are inversely associated with breast cancer risk among Chinese women: A case-control study. *British Journal of Nutrition* 15 (1): 129–37.

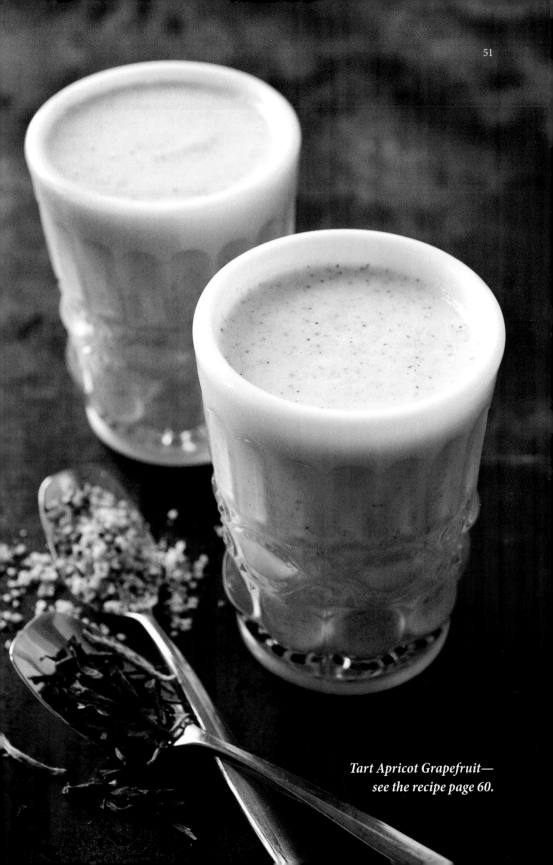

Tart Apricot Grapefruit—
see the recipe page 60.

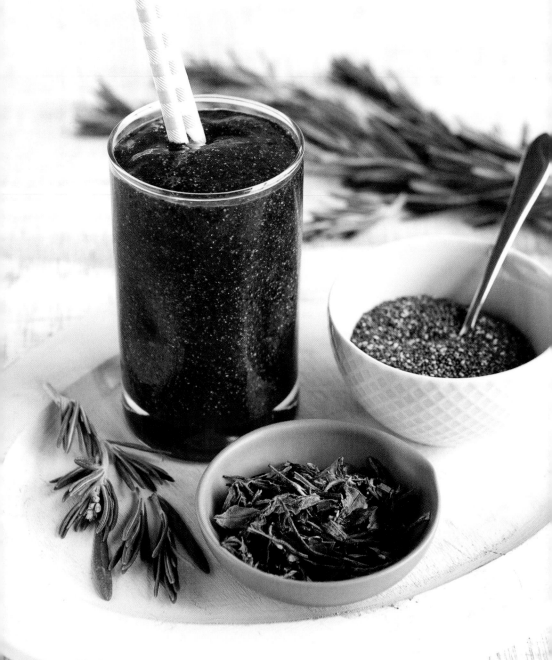

Wild Blueberry and Spiced Apple—see the recipe page 65.

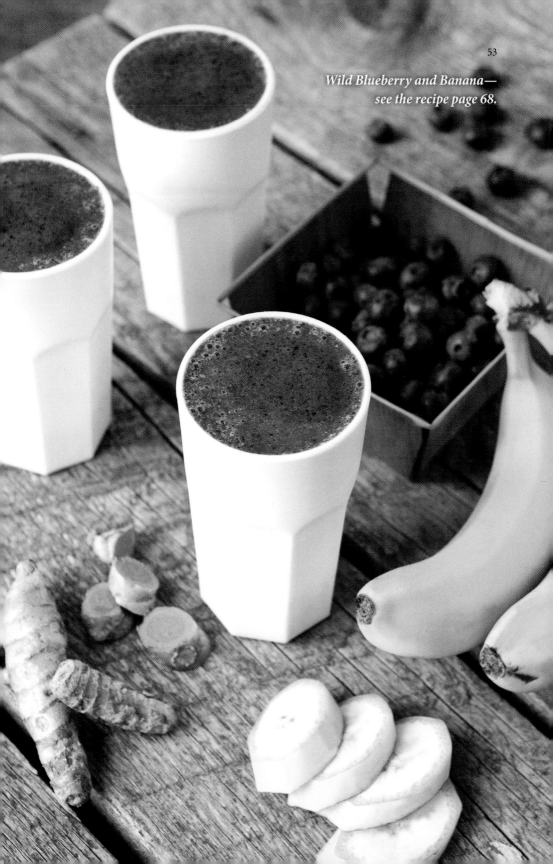

Wild Blueberry and Banana—
see the recipe page 68.

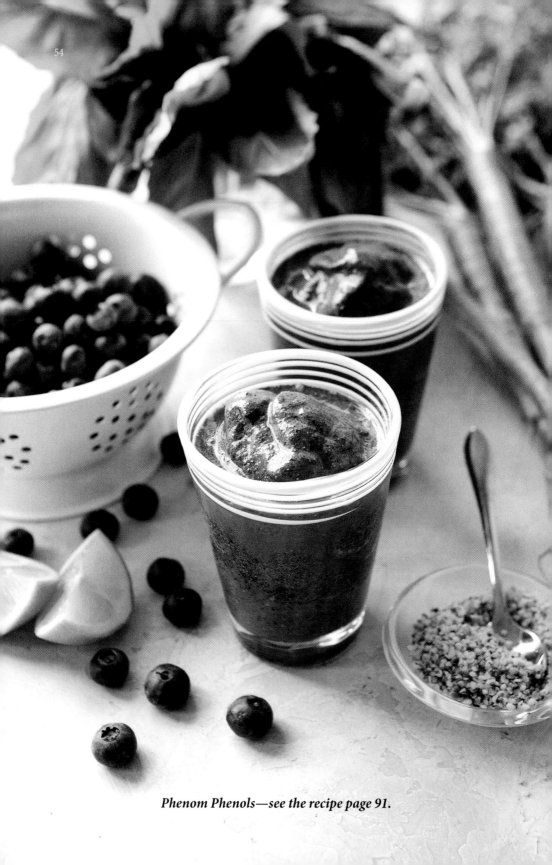

Phenom Phenols—see the recipe page 91.

HERBAL APRICOT

*R*ich apricot is the predominant flavor in this light and aromatic blend.

Apricots contain antioxidants that can reduce precancerous cell changes that may lead to the formation of breast tumors. In a study of postmenopausal breast cancer survivors, a significant association was found between higher blood carotenoid levels and lower numbers of cell markers of oxidative stress.

SERVES ❷

1 apricot
1 cup apricot nectar
½ cup green tea ice cubes
¼ cup fresh basil leaves
¼ cup hulled hemp seed
Pinch of turmeric powder

Combine all ingredients in a high-power blender or food processor and blend until smooth. Drink immediately.

Nutrition Facts *(per serving)*

Calories 210; Fat 9; Protein 9; Carbs 22; Fiber 4; Net Carbs 18

Research Study

C. A. Thomson, N. R. Stendell-Hollis, C. L. Rock, et al. (2007). Plasma and dietary carotenoids are associated with reduced oxidative stress in women previously treated for breast cancer. *Cancer Epidemiology, Biomarkers and Prevention* 16 (10): 2008–15.

GOLDEN APRICOT PLUM

*T*his rich plum and apricot smoothie has a golden color and green tea fragrance.

Lycopene, found in concentration in apricots, exhibits anticancer action via its high antioxidant capacity, which has been demonstrated in both in vitro and in vivo tumor models. Lycopene selectively arrests cell growth and induces apoptosis in cancer cells without affecting normal cells.

SERVES **2**

2 plums

1 cup apricot nectar

½ cup green tea ice cubes

¼ cup hulled hemp seed

½ teaspoon turmeric powder

Combine all ingredients in a high-power blender or food processor and blend until smooth. Drink immediately.

Nutrition Facts *(per serving)*

Calories 210; Fat 9; Protein 8; Carbs 23; Fiber 3; Net Carbs 20

Research Study

C. Trejo-Solís, J. Pedraza-Chaverrí, M. Torres-Ramos, et al. (2013). Multiple molecular and cellular mechanisms of action of lycopene in cancer inhibition. *Evidence-Based Complementary and Alternative Medicine*, article ID 705121.

CHERRY APRICOT FROSTY

*T*his frosty and slightly sweet smoothie is rich in cherry flavor.

Apricot compounds, such as oleanolic and ursolic acid, have been found to suppress breast cancer cells in laboratory studies.

SERVES ❷

1 cup frozen cherries

½ cup apricot nectar

½ cup green tea ice cubes

2 tablespoons hulled hemp seed

½ teaspoon turmeric power

Combine all ingredients in a high-power blender or food processor and blend until smooth. Drink immediately.

Nutrition Facts *(per serving)*

Calories 100; Fat 5; Protein 8; Carbs 12; Fiber 1; Net Carbs 11

Research Study

M. Hattori, K. Kawakami, M. Akimoto, et al. (2013). Antitumor effect of Japanese apricot extract (MK615) on human cancer cells in vitro and in vivo through a reactive oxygen species-dependent mechanism. *Tumori* 99 (2): 239–48.

CITRUS BERRY PUNCH

This luscious, fruity combination is light and sweet and has a creamy texture from the blended hemp seed.

Grape skin polyphenols have been found to successfully inhibit the spread of breast cancer cells. When grape skin extracts were tested on human cells and in mice, they significantly reduced metastases and triggered apoptosis.

SERVES ❷

1 cup frozen grapes

½ cup apricot nectar

½ cup frozen strawberries

¼ cup hulled hemp seed

2 teaspoons lime juice

Combine all ingredients in a high-power blender or food processor and blend until smooth. Drink immediately.

Nutrition Facts *(per serving)*

Calories 180; Fat 9; Protein 7; Carbs 20; Fiber 3; Net Carbs 17

Research Study

T. Sun, Q. Y. Chen, L. J. Wu, et al. (2012). Antitumor and antimetastatic activities of grape skin polyphenols in a murine model of breast cancer. *Food and Chemical Toxicology* 64 (9): 609–14.

LYCOPENE LUSTER

*W*atermelon is not only rich in cancer-fighting carotenoids, but it also sweetens vegetable smoothies.

Carotenoids, found in both tomatoes and watermelon, act as antioxidants, reducing free radicals in the body, and they are especially protective against invasive breast cancer in premenopausal women. Since free radicals are a precursor of cancerous cells, they protect the body from developing cancer and also reduce tumor growth.

SERVES ❷

1 tomato

1 cup watermelon

½ cup apricot nectar

½ cup greens

¼ cup hulled hemp seed

Combine all ingredients in a high-power blender or food processor and blend until smooth. Drink immediately.

Nutrition Facts *(per serving)*

Calories 180; Fat 9; Protein 6; Carbs 18; Fiber 2; Net Carbs 16

Research Study

L. I. Mignone, E. Giovannucci, P. A. Newcomb, et al. (2009). Dietary carotenoids and the risk of invasive breast cancer. *International Journal of Cancer* 124 (12): 2929–37.

TART APRICOT GRAPEFRUIT

*T*his intense and creamy grapefruit smoothie has a bit of healthy, nutty flavor from the hemp seed. See photo page 51.

Nobiletin is a bioflavonoid found in citrus fruits, such as lemons, oranges, tangerines, and grapefruits. The most-studied properties of nobiletin are its anti-inflammatory and anticancer activities. This nutrient has an epigenetic effect with potential to suppress metastasis of breast cancer.
Apricot and grapefruit also provide breast cancer protective carotenoids.

SERVES ❷

1 apricot
½ cup grapefruit juice
½ cup green tea ice cubes
¼ cup hulled hemp seed

Combine all ingredients in a high-power blender or food processor and blend until smooth. Drink immediately.

Nutrition Facts *(per serving)*
Calories 150; Fat 9; Protein 7; Carbs 10; Fiber 2; Net Carbs 8

Research Study
S. H. Baek, S. M. Kim, D. Nam, et al. (2012). Antimetastatic effect of nobiletin through the down-regulation of CXC chemokine receptor type 4 and matrix metallopeptidase-9. *Pharmaceutical Biology* 50 (10): 1210–18.

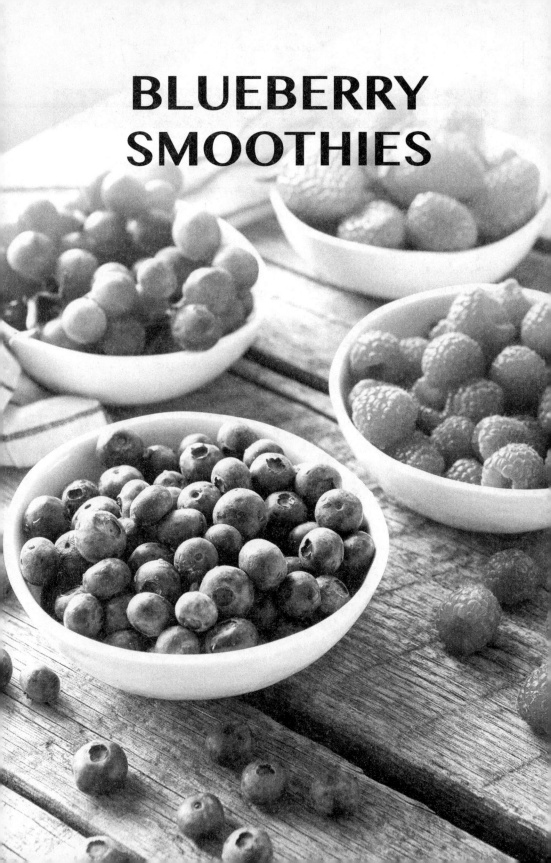

BLUEBERRY SMOOTHIES

BLUEBERRY CHERRY

*T*hick and frosty with strong mango and cherry flavors, this delicious combination could be served as a dessert.

Pterostilbene, a natural compound isolated from blueberries, effectively suppresses potential breast cancer stem cells in laboratory studies.

SERVES ❸

½ cup wild blueberries

½ cup blueberry nectar

½ cup frozen mango

½ cup frozen cherries

½ cup green tea

¼ cup hulled hemp seed

½ teaspoon turmeric powder

Combine all ingredients in a high-power blender or food processor and blend until smooth. Drink immediately.

Nutrition Facts *(per serving)*

Calories 130; Fat 6; Protein 5; Carbs 20; Fiber 2; Net Carbs 18

Research Study

K. K. Mak, A. T. Wu, W. H. Lee, et al. (2013). Pterostilbene, a bioactive component of blueberries, suppresses the generation of breast cancer stem cells within tumor microenvironment and metastasis via modulating NF-κB/microRNA 448 circuit. *Molecular Nutrition and Food Research* 57 (7): 1123–34.

BLUE WATERMELON POM

This summer fruit combination is light and slightly creamy with concentrated pomegranate flavor.

Pomegranate fruit is rich in antioxidant tannins and flavonoids that inhibit the growth of breast cancer cells in culture.

SERVES ❶

1 cup green tea ice cubes

½ cup blueberry nectar

½ cup watermelon

½ cup pomegranate juice

¼ cup hulled hemp seed

2 teaspoons lemon juice

Combine all ingredients in a high-power blender or food processor and blend until smooth. Drink immediately.

Nutrition Facts *(per serving)*

Calories 130; Fat 6; Protein 5; Carbs 14; Fiber 1; Net Carbs 13

Research Study

V. M. Adhami, N. Khan, and H. Mukhtar. (2009). Cancer chemoprevention by pomegranate: Laboratory and clinical evidence. *Nutrition and Cancer* 61 (6): 811–15.

RASPBERRY LIME

This deep red drink is creamy, slightly tart, and rich in berry flavor.

Raspberries contain carotenoids, vitamin C, and anthocyanins, which worked together to decrease the growth and spread of breast cancer cells in laboratory studies. A large-scale cohort study found that high vegetable intake is associated with a lower risk of hormone receptor–negative breast cancer.

SERVES ❷

1 cup green tea ice cubes

½ cup blueberry nectar

½ cup watermelon

½ cup frozen raspberries

¼ cup hulled hemp seed

1 teaspoon lime juice

Combine all ingredients in a high-power blender or food processor and blend until smooth. Drink immediately.

Nutrition Facts *(per serving)*

Calories 182; Fat 6; Protein 6; Carbs 22; Fiber 2; Net Carbs 20

Research Study

M. J. Emaus, P. H. Peeters, M. F. Bakker, et al. (2016). Vegetable and fruit consumption and the risk of hormone receptor-defined breast cancer in the EPIC cohort. *American Journal of Clinical Nutrition* 103 (1): 168–77.

WILD BLUEBERRY AND SPICED APPLE

A rich and flavorful blend of apple and wild blueberries, this smoothie has complex spice flavors and fragrance. See photo page 52.

Black pepper and cardamom are spices that in combination help regulate inflammation by suppressing pro-inflammatory immune cells and may also help the immune system fight cancer. Imbalances in the immune system can lead to excess inflammation, which can cause damage to cells, leading to abnormal mutations. By helping to regulate the inflammatory response, these spices may reduce the risk of cancer and help fight existing cancer cells.

SERVES ❷

1 cup frozen wild blueberries

½ cup unfiltered apple juice

½ cup green tea ice cubes

2 tablespoons protein powder

2 tablespoons chia seed

¼ teaspoon turmeric powder

¼ teaspoon cardamom powder

Pinch of fresh ground black pepper

Combine all ingredients in a high-power blender or food processor and blend until smooth. Drink immediately.

Nutrition Facts *(per serving)*

Calories 200; Fat 7; Protein 11; Carbs 26; Fiber 11; Net Carbs 15

Research Study

A. F. Majdalawieh and R. I. Carr. (2010). In vitro investigation of the potential immunomodulatory and anticancer activities of black pepper *(Piper nigrum)* and cardamom *(Elettaria cardamomum). Journal of Medicinal Food* 13 (2): 371–81.

HOT GINGER AND BLUEBERRY

*T*his luxurious blueberry smoothie has a hot ginger bite and light green tea base.

Ginger contains anticancer nutrients, such as shogaol, which are showing potential as therapeutic and preventive agents. Ginger root also provides vanilloids that possess anti-inflammatory and anticancer properties.

SERVES ❸

1 cup wild blueberries

1 cup blueberry nectar

1 cup green tea ice cubes

¼ cup hulled hemp seed

1 tablespoon fresh ginger root

Combine all ingredients in a high-power blender or food processor and blend until smooth. Drink immediately.

Nutrition Facts *(per serving)*

Calories 140; Fat 6; Protein 5; Carbs 17; Fiber 2; Net Carbs 15

Research Study

F. F. Gan, H. Ling, X. Ang, et al. (2013). A novel shogaol analog suppresses cancer cell invasion and inflammation, and displays cytoprotective effects through modulation of NF-κB and Nrf2-Keap1 signaling pathways. *Toxicology and Applied Pharmacology* 272 (3): 852–62.

BASIL BERRY BLEND

*T*his rich berry combination has a fresh basil scent and blueberry flavor.

Blueberry phytochemicals inhibit the growth and metastatic potential of breast cancer cells and have a preventive effect on triple-negative breast cancer.

SERVES ❷

½ cup fresh basil leaves

½ cup frozen wild blueberries

½ cup blueberry nectar

½ cup green tea ice cubes

2 tablespoons chia seed

Combine all ingredients in a high-power blender or food processor and blend until smooth. Drink immediately.

Nutrition Facts *(per serving)*

Calories 120; Fat 5; Protein 4; Carbs 18; Fiber 7; Net Carbs 11

Research Study

L. S. Adams, S. Phung, N. Yee, et al. (2010). Blueberry phytochemicals inhibit growth and metastatic potential of MDA-MB-231 breast cancer cells through modulation of the phosphatidylinositol 3-kinase pathway. *Cancer Research* 70 (9): 3594–605.

WILD BLUEBERRY AND BANANA

This smoothie has potent blueberry and banana flavors and a gorgeous purple hue (see photo page 53).

Curcumin, found in turmeric, and the omega fatty acids found in hulled hemp seed, both provide anti-inflammatory action that protects against inflammation-induced fatigue in cancer patients and those in remission.

SERVES ❷

1 cup frozen wild blueberries

1 cup green tea ice cubes

½ banana

¼ cup hulled hemp seed

1 teaspoon lemon juice

½ teaspoon turmeric powder

Combine all ingredients in a high-power blender or food processor and blend until smooth. Drink immediately.

Nutrition Facts *(per serving)*

Calories 210; Fat 9; Protein 8; Carbs 25; Fiber 5; Net Carbs 20

Research Study

C. M. Alfano, I. Imayama, M. L. Neuhouser, et al. (2012). Fatigue, inflammation, and ω-3 and ω-6 fatty acid intake among breast cancer survivors. *Journal of Clinical Oncology* 30 (12): 1280–87.

WILD BLUEBERRY AND MANGO

This berry and mango combination is the perfect balance of sweet and tart flavors.

A diet rich in mango, papaya, and avocado appears to reduce the risk of development of breast cancer.

SERVES ❷

½ cup frozen wild blueberries

½ cup blueberry nectar

½ cup frozen mango

½ cup green tea ice cubes

2 tablespoons chia seed

2 tablespoons protein powder

Combine all ingredients in a high-power blender or food processor and blend until smooth. Drink immediately.

Nutrition Facts *(per serving)*

Calories 200; Fat 7; Protein 11; Carbs 27; Fiber 11; Net Carbs 16

Research Study

I. Jordan, A. Hebestreit, B. Swai, et al. (2013). Dietary patterns and breast cancer risk among women in northern Tanzania: A case-control study. *European Journal of Nutrition* 52 (3): 905–15.

BLUEBERRY ORANGE

*T*his simple combination is sweet, protein-rich, and full of citrus and berry flavors.

Naringin, a flavonoid extracted from citrus fruits such as oranges, appears to inhibit the growth potential of triple-negative (ER-/PR-/HER2-) breast cancer (TNBC).

SERVES ❷

1 orange

1 cup white tea

½ cup blueberry nectar

¼ cup hulled hemp seed

Combine all ingredients in a high-power blender or food processor and blend until smooth. Drink immediately.

Nutrition Facts *(per serving)*

Calories 180; Fat 9; Protein 7; Carbs 17; Fiber 3; Net Carbs 14

Research Study

H. Li, B. Yang, J. Huang, et al. (2013). Naringin inhibits growth potential of human triple-negative breast cancer cells by targeting β-catenin signaling pathway. *Toxicology Letters* 220 (3): 219–28.

STRAWBERRY HEMP SHAKE

This blend has vivid berry color and flavor, is slightly sweet, and has just a hint of green tea.

Epigallocatechin-gallate (EGCG) is a major biologically active component of green tea. Romanian researchers found that EGCG suppresses the growth, migration, and invasion of human breast cancer cells by changing human breast cancer cell gene expression.

SERVES ❷

½ cup blueberry nectar

½ cup green tea ice cubes

½ cup wild blueberries

½ cup frozen strawberries

¼ cup hulled hemp seed

Combine all ingredients in a high-power blender or food processor and blend until smooth. Drink immediately.

Nutrition Facts *(per serving)*

Calories 170; Fat 9; Protein 7; Carbs 16; Fiber 3; Net Carbs 13

Research Study

C. Braicu, C. D. Gherman, A. Irimie, et al. (2013). Epigallocatechin-gallate (EGCG) inhibits cell proliferation and migratory behavior of triple negative breast cancer cells. *Journal of Nanoscience and Nanotechnology* 13 (1): 632–37.

BERRY BURST FROSTY

*T*his lush and pink raspberry and cherry combination is creamy from the hemp and has an intense flavor with a tart edge.

Ellagic acid, found in raspberries, is chemopreventive in breast cancer development.

SERVES ❷

½ cup blueberry nectar

½ cup frozen raspberries

½ cup frozen cherries

½ cup water

¼ cup hulled hemp seed

Combine all ingredients in a high-power blender or food processor and blend until smooth. Drink immediately.

Nutrition Facts *(per serving)*

Calories 160; Fat 9; Protein 7; Carbs 15; Fiber 2; Net Carbs 13

Research Study

R. Munagala, F. Aqil, M. V. Vadhanam, et al. (2013). MicroRNA "signature" during estrogen-mediated mammary carcinogenesis and its reversal by ellagic acid intervention. *Cancer Letters* 339 (2): 175–84.

WILD BLUEBERRY AND GREEN TEA

This smoothie delivers wild blueberry flavor and color with a light sweetness that is mellowed by green tea.

Epigallocatechin-gallate (EGCG), a green tea catechin, has preventive and inhibitory effects on the growth of existing breast cancer tumors.

SERVES ❷

1 cup frozen wild blueberries

½ cup green tea ice cubes

½ cup blueberry nectar

¼ cup chia seed

Combine all ingredients in a high-power blender or food processor and blend until smooth. Drink immediately.

Nutrition Facts *(per serving)*

Calories 210; Fat 11; Protein 7; Carbs 28; Fiber 14; Net Carbs 14

Research Study

M. Donejko, M. Niczyporuk, E. Galicka, et al. (2013). Anticancer properties epigallocatechin-gallate contained in green tea. *Postępy higieny i medycyny doświadczalnej* (Online) 67:26–34.

WILD BLUEBERRY AND RASPBERRY

*T*his berry combination is sorbet-like, thick, and frosty with a bit of citrus.

Daily intake of green tea has been found to provide enough epigallocatechin-gallate (EGCG), to reduce growth and spread of breast cancer cells and to induce apoptosis and decrease growth of preexisting inflammatory breast cancer (IBC) cells and tumors.

SERVES ❸

1 cup green tea ice cubes

½ cup frozen wild blueberries

½ cup raspberries

½ cup blueberry nectar

¼ cup hulled hemp seed

1 teaspoon lemon juice

Combine all ingredients in a high-power blender or food processor and blend until smooth. Drink immediately.

Nutrition Facts *(per serving)*

Calories 120; Fat 6; Protein 5; Carbs 11; Fiber 3; Net Carbs 8

Research Study

N. D. Mineva, K. E. Paulson, S. P. Naber, et al. (2013). Epigallocatechin-gallate inhibits stem-like inflammatory breast cancer cells. *PLoS One* 8 (9): e73464.

CARNOSIC BERRY

This blend has rich blueberry tang and complex basil and tea flavors.

Rosemary contains carnosic acid, which displays significant growth inhibitory activity on breast cancer cells. Carnosic acid activates apoptosis and suppresses the expression of genes involved in cancer cell development in laboratory studies. Researchers believe carnosic acid from rosemary may prevent and even treat estrogen receptor negative (ER-) breast cancer. These effects are amplified when carnosic acid is combined with curcumin (from turmeric).

SERVES ❶

1 cup green tea ice cubes

½ cup frozen blueberries

2 tablespoons hulled hemp seed

¼ teaspoon rosemary leaf powder

¼ teaspoon turmeric powder

Combine all ingredients in a high-power blender or food processor and blend until smooth. Drink immediately.

Nutrition Facts *(per serving)*

Calories 140; Fat 9; Protein 7; Carbs 11; Fiber 5; Net Carbs 6

Research Study

L. S. Einbond, H. A. Wu, R. Kashiwazaki, et al. (2012). Carnosic acid inhibits the growth of ER-negative human breast cancer cells and synergizes with curcumin. *Fitoterapia* 83 (7): 1160–68.

WILD BLUEBERRY PINEAPPLE

*S*imultaneously light and rich, this blueberry and pineapple combination is just slightly sweet.

Bromelain, a proteolytic enzyme from pineapple, triggers autophagy and apoptosis (self-destruction) of breast cancer cells.

SERVES ❷

1 cup cultured coconut milk

½ cup frozen wild blueberries

½ cup frozen pineapple

2 tablespoons hulled hemp seed

Combine all ingredients in a high-power blender or food processor and blend until smooth. Drink immediately.

Nutrition Facts *(per serving)*

Calories 180; Fat 7; Protein 6; Carbs 15; Fiber 4; Net Carbs 11

Research Study

K. Bhui, S. Tyagi, B. Prakash, et al. (2010). Pineapple bromelain induces autophagy, facilitating apoptotic response in mammary carcinoma cells. *BioFactors* 36 (6): 474–82.

HOLY BASIL ELIXIR

*C*ool and light, this wild blueberry and green tea blend has fresh basil and lime flavors.

Extracts from holy basil (tulsi) have shown anticancer activity, such as inhibition of tumor growth in laboratory studies.

SERVES ❷

1 cup green tea ice cubes

½ cup fresh holy basil leaves

½ cup frozen wild blueberries

½ cup coconut water

¼ cup hulled hemp seed

2 teaspoons lime juice

Combine all ingredients in a high-power blender or food processor and blend until smooth. Drink immediately.

Nutrition Facts *(per serving)*

Calories 180; Fat 5; Protein 4; Carbs 6; Fiber 2; Net Carbs 4

Research Study

P. Nangia-Makker, T. Raz, L. Tait, et al. (2013). Ocimum gratissimum retards breast cancer growth and progression and is a natural inhibitor of matrix metalloproteases. *Cancer Biology and Therapy* 14 (5): 417–27.

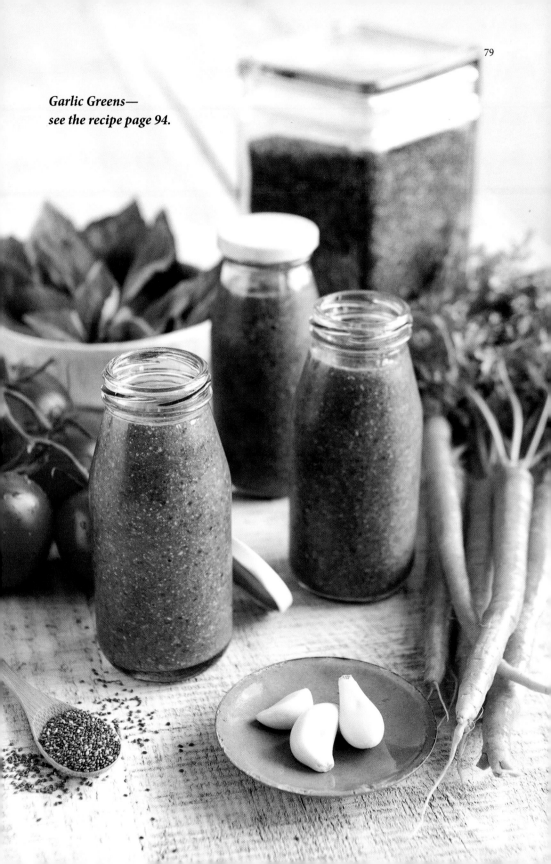

Garlic Greens—
see the recipe page 94.

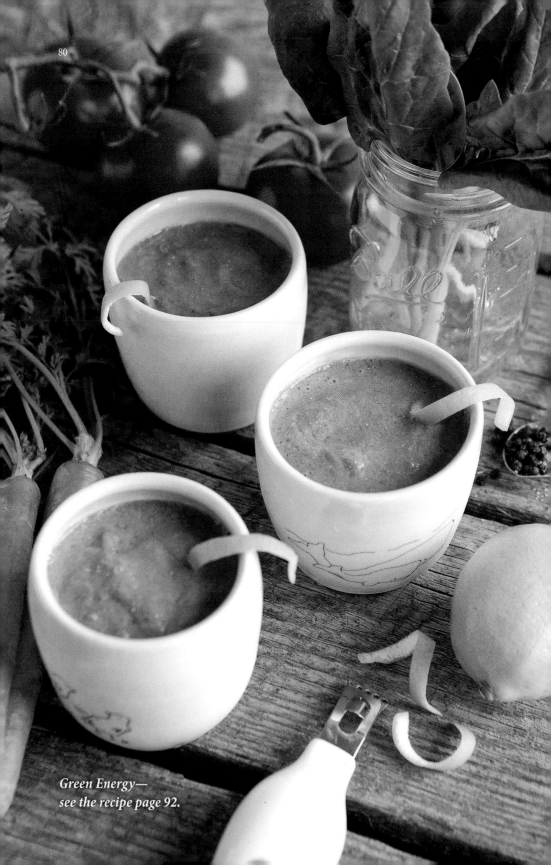

Green Energy—
see the recipe page 92.

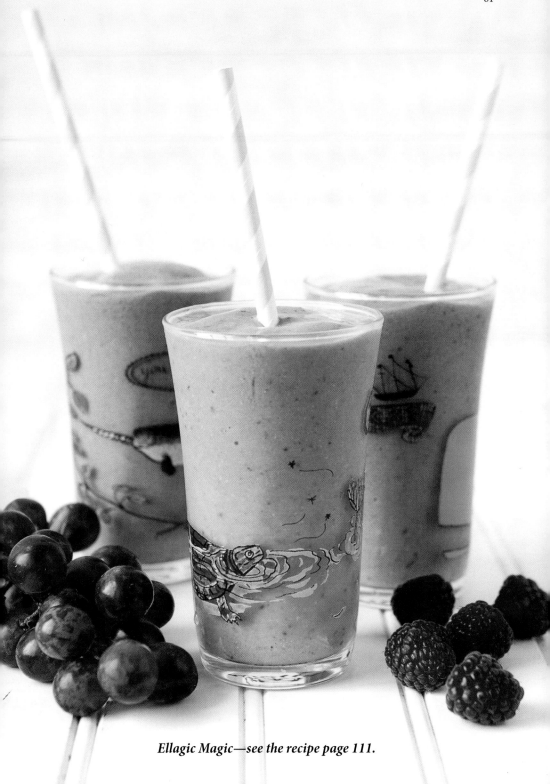

Ellagic Magic—see the recipe page 111.

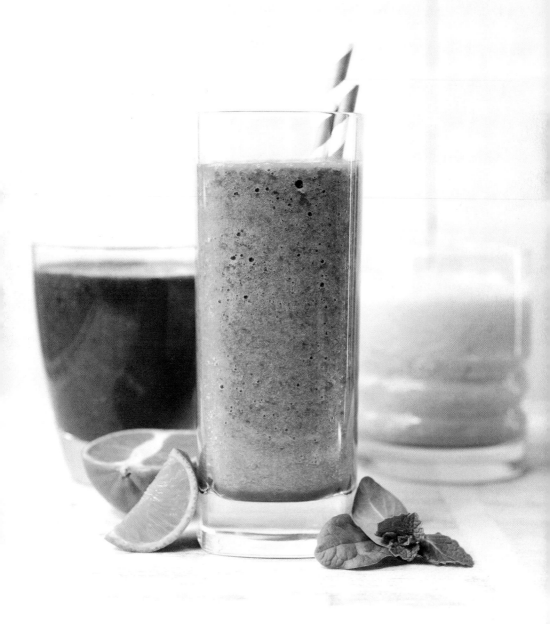

*Add a variety of whole plant foods to your smoothies to ensure
your daily diet is filled with a wide range of nutrients.*

CARROT JUICE SMOOTHIES

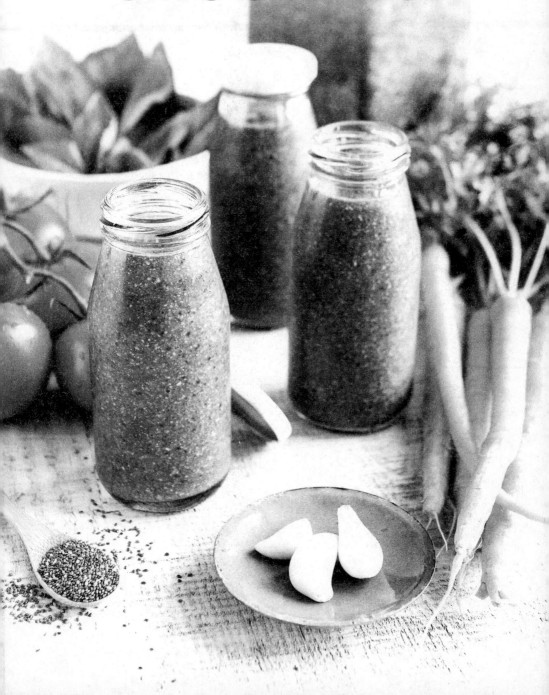

PINEAPPLE CARROT

*T*his creamy pineapple combination has fresh carrot flavor with a hint of rosemary, and it packs a punch of protein.

Rosemary contains carnosol, carnosic acid, ursolic acid, and rosmarinic acid, which have been found to suppress the development of breast tumors.

SERVES ❷

½ cup carrot juice

½ cup frozen pineapple

¼ cup hulled hemp seed

2 teaspoons lime juice

½ teaspoon rosemary leaf powder

Combine all ingredients in a high-power blender or food processor and blend until smooth. Drink immediately.

Nutrition Facts *(per serving)*

Calories 160; Fat 9; Protein 8; Carbs 13; Fiber 3; Net Carbs 10

Research Study

S. N. Ngo, D. B. Williams, and R. J. Head. (2011). Rosemary and cancer prevention: Preclinical perspectives. *Critical Reviews in Food Science and Nutrition* 51 (10): 946–54.

STRAWBERRY CARROT BASIL

*T*his sweet and herbal combination is unusual and delicious. It's frosty, aromatic, and addictive!

Basil contains eugenol, which exhibits inhibition of breast cancer cells by reducing their growth and triggering apoptosis. This was determined by microscopic examination of eugenol-treated cells, showing cell shrinkage, membrane breakdown, and apoptotic body formation.

SERVES ❷

½ cup carrot juice

½ cup frozen strawberries

½ cup fresh basil leaves

½ cup green tea ice cubes

2 tablespoons chia seed

¼ teaspoon turmeric powder

Combine all ingredients in a high-power blender or food processor and blend until smooth. Drink immediately.

Nutrition Facts *(per serving)*

Calories 110; Fat 6; Protein 4; Carbs 15; Fiber 8; Net Carbs 7

Research Study

N. Vidhya and S. N. Devaraj. (2011). Induction of apoptosis by eugenol in human breast cancer cells. *Indian Journal of Experimental Biology* 49 (11): 871–78.

CARROT AND CITRUS

*C*ool and refreshing, this flavorful combination is slightly sweet with a hint of citrus.

Both carrots and kale contain carotenoids, which are antioxidants that can reduce precancerous cell changes and reduce breast cancer cell growth. Dietary carotenoids (alpha-carotene and beta-carotene) reduce the risk of ER-/PR- breast cancer (see "hormone sensitive" in the Glossary of Terms), even among smokers.

SERVES ❷

1 cup carrot juice

1 cup green tea ice cubes

½ cup kale

2 tablespoons chia seed

1 tablespoon lemon juice

¼ teaspoon turmeric powder

Pinch of fresh ground black pepper

Combine all ingredients in a high-power blender or food processor and blend until smooth. Drink immediately.

Nutrition Facts *(per serving)*

Calories 120; Fat 5; Protein 4; Carbs 17; Fiber 7; Net Carbs 10

Research Studies

S. C. Larsson, L. Bergkvist, and A. Wolk. (2010). Dietary carotenoids and risk of hormone receptor-defined breast cancer in a prospective cohort of Swedish women. *European Journal of Cancer* 46 (6): 1079–85.

R. M. Tamimi, G. A. Colditz, and S. E. Hankinson. (2009). Circulating carotenoids, mammographic density, and subsequent risk of breast cancer. *Cancer Prevention Research* 69 (24): 9323–29.

CITRUS BEET

A *cool, frosty, deep red vegetable blend that has an earthy turmeric scent and a hint of lemon.*

Beets contain antioxidant carotenoids, and higher carotenoid levels in the blood are linked to lower numbers of breast cancer cells. Eating beets boosts carotenoid blood levels, which provides cellular protection against oxidative damage particularly among women with a high mammographic density.

SERVES ❷

1 cup green tea ice cubes

½ cup carrot juice

½ cup raw beet

½ cup spinach

1 tablespoon lemon juice

¼ teaspoon turmeric powder

Pinch of fresh ground black pepper

Combine all ingredients in a high-power blender or food processor and blend until smooth. Drink immediately.

Nutrition Facts *(per serving)*

Calories 25; Fat 0; Protein 1; Carbs 6; Fiber 1; Net Carbs 5

Research Study

A. H. Eliassen, X. Liao, B. Rosner, et al. (2015). Plasma carotenoids and risk of breast cancer over 20 years of follow-up. *American Journal of Clinical Nutrition* 101 (6): 1197–205.

GARLIC IMMUNE CHARGER

*C*arrot juice gives this frosty combination a sweet vegetable base, while garlic gives it a hot and spicy kick!

Sulfur compounds, such as diallyl trisulfide in garlic, appear to inhibit breast tumor growth by inducing apoptosis (cancer cell death). Garlic contains strong-smelling organosulfur compounds, some of which are shown to reduce the growth and spread of tumors in laboratory studies.

SERVES ❶

½ cup carrot juice

½ cup green tea ice cubes

2 tablespoons chia seed

1 clove garlic

1 tablespoon lemon juice

¼ teaspoon turmeric powder

Combine all ingredients in a high-power blender or food processor and blend until smooth. Drink immediately.

Nutrition Facts *(per serving)*

Calories 190; Fat 10; Protein 7; Carbs 23; Fiber 13; Net Carbs 10

Research Study

K. Chandra-Kuntal, J. Lee, and S. V. Singh. (2013). Critical role for reactive oxygen species in apoptosis induction and cell migration inhibition by diallyl trisulfide, a cancer chemopreventive component of garlic. *Breast Cancer Treatment and Research* 138 (1): 69–79.

CARROT CILANTRO

This slightly sweet blend has the perfect balance of sweet and savory with a touch of fresh lemon.

Fresh extracts of garlic arrested the growth of breast cancer cells in laboratory studies.
A large-scale cohort study found that high vegetable intake is associated with lower hormone receptor–negative breast cancer risk.

SERVES ❷

½ cup carrot juice

½ cup green tea ice cubes

½ cup spinach

¼ cup fresh cilantro

2 tablespoons hulled hemp seed

2 teaspoons lemon juice

¼ teaspoon turmeric powder

Combine all ingredients in a high-power blender or food processor and blend until smooth. Drink immediately.

Nutrition Facts *(per serving)*

Calories 160; Fat 9; Protein 8; Carbs 14; Fiber 3; Net Carbs 11

Research Studies

S. Modem, S. E. Dicarlo, and T. R. Reddy. (2012). Fresh garlic extract induces growth arrest and morphological differentiation of MCF7 breast cancer cells. *Genes and Cancer* 3 (2): 177–86.

M. J. Emaus, P. H. Peeters, M. F. Bakker, et al. (2016). Vegetable and fruit consumption and the risk of hormone receptor-defined breast cancer in the EPIC cohort. *American Journal of Clinical Nutrition* 103 (1): 168–77.

CARROT MANGO CHERRY

*T*his creamy mango and carrot smoothie is slightly sweet with a hint of
tartness.

Carotenoid antioxidants found in carrots reduce oxidative stress, which provides breast cancer protection, especially for those who are postmenopausal or ER+.

SERVES ❸

1 cup carrot juice

1 cup coconut water

½ cup frozen mango

½ cup frozen cherries

¼ cup hulled hemp seed

2 teaspoons lemon juice

Combine all ingredients in a high-power blender or food processor and blend until smooth. Drink immediately.

Nutrition Facts *(per serving)*

Calories 150; Fat 6; Protein 5; Carbs 18; Fiber 2; Net Carbs 16

Research Study

Y. Wang, S. M. Gapstur, M. M. Gaudet, et al. (2015). Plasma carotenoids and breast cancer risk in the Cancer Prevention Study II Nutrition Cohort. *Cancer Causes & Control* 26 (9): 1233–44.

PHENOM PHENOLS

*T*his bright purple smoothie (see photo page 54) has fresh basil flavor and fragrance.

Curcumin was shown to reduce insulin-like growth factor, which is important as higher levels of insulin-like growth factor are associated with increased breast cancer diagnoses.

SERVES ❷

½ cup carrot juice

½ cup wild blueberries

½ cup green tea ice cubes

½ cup fresh basil leaves

2 tablespoons hulled hemp seed

2 teaspoons lemon juice

½ teaspoon turmeric powder

Combine all ingredients in a high-power blender or food processor and blend until smooth. Drink immediately.

Nutrition Facts *(per serving)*

Calories 100; Fat 5; Protein 5; Carbs 11; Fiber 2; Net Carbs 9

Research Study

Y. Xia, L. Jin, B. Zhang, et al. (2007). The potentiation of curcumin on insulin-like growth factor-1 action in MCF-7 human breast carcinoma cells. *Life Sciences* 80 (23): 2161–69.

GREEN ENERGY

*T*his cool, green smoothie (see photo page 80) has fresh vegetable and citrus flavors.

Carrots, tomatoes, and greens are all rich in carotenoids, which reduce cellular oxidation, a biological precursor to breast cancer. Studies have found that women with higher blood levels of alpha-carotene, beta-carotene, lycopene, lutein, and zeaxanthin may have a reduced risk of breast cancer.

SERVES ❷

1 tomato

½ cup carrot juice

½ cup greens

½ cup green tea ice cubes

¼ cup hulled hemp seed

1 tablespoon lemon juice

Pinch of fresh ground black pepper

Pinch of turmeric

Combine all ingredients in a high-power blender or food processor and blend until smooth. Drink immediately.

Nutrition Facts *(per serving)*

Calories 140; Fat 9; Protein 7; Carbs 8; Fiber 2; Net Carbs 6

Research Study

A. H. Eliassen, S. J. Hendrickson, L. A. Brinton, et al. (2012). Circulating carotenoids and risk of breast cancer: Pooled analysis of eight prospective studies. *Journal of the National Cancer Institute* 104 (24): 1905–16.

ROSEMARY CARROT COOLER

*C*arrot juice gives this blend a fresh flavor while the green tea and rosemary lend delicate, aromatic layers.

Rosemary leaf is a rich source of carnosol, which supports the reduction of inflammation as well as triggering apoptosis of breast cancer cells.

SERVES ❶

1 cup green tea ice cubes

½ cup carrot juice

2 tablespoons chia seed

1 teaspoon lemon juice

½ teaspoon rosemary leaf powder

Combine all ingredients in a high-power blender or food processor and blend until smooth. Drink immediately.

Nutrition Facts *(per serving)*

Calories 190; Fat 10; Protein 7; Carbs 23; Fiber 13; Net Carbs 10

Research Study

J. J. Johnson. (2011). Carnosol: A promising anticancer and anti-inflammatory agent. *Cancer Letters* 305 (1): 1–7.

GARLIC GREENS

*T*he fresh vegetable flavor in this smoothie hits the palate first and finishes with a little hot garlic bite. See photo page 79.

A review of several European studies found that those who eat garlic regularly have a lower risk for breast cancer. In addition, diallyl disulphide, an organosulfur compound in garlic, has been found to lower the incidence of breast cancer via apoptosis.

SERVES ❷

½ cup carrot juice

½ cup tomato

½ cup greens

½ cup green tea ice cubes

2 tablespoons chia seed

1 clove raw garlic

Pinch of fresh ground black pepper

Combine all ingredients in a high-power blender or food processor and blend until smooth. Drink immediately.

Nutrition Facts *(per serving)*

Calories 100; Fat 5; Protein 4; Carbs 14; Fiber 7; Net Carbs 7

Research Study

M. O. Altonsy, T. N. Habib, and S. C. Andrews. (2012). Diallyl disulfide-induced apoptosis in a breast-cancer cell line (MCF-7) may be caused by inhibition of histone deacetylation. *Nutrition and Cancer* 64 (8): 1251–60.

CAROTENOID QUEEN

*T*his smoothie has fresh vegetable flavor with a bit of sweet and frosty mango.

Increasing plasma (blood) carotenoid concentrations by eating carotenoid-rich foods, such as carrots and mango, reduces the risk for breast cancer recurrence.

SERVES ❷

½ cup carrot juice

½ cup fresh holy basil leaves

½ cup frozen mango

½ cup green tea ice cubes

2 tablespoons hulled hemp seed

Combine all ingredients in a high-power blender or food processor and blend until smooth. Drink immediately.

Nutrition Facts *(per serving)*

Calories 115; Fat 5; Protein 4; Carbs 15; Fiber 2; Net Carbs 13

Research Study

C. L. Rock, S. W. Flatt, L. Natarajan, et al. (2005). Plasma carotenoids and recurrence-free survival in women with a history of breast cancer. *Journal of Clinical Oncology* 23 (27): 6631–38.

COCONUT WATER SMOOTHIES

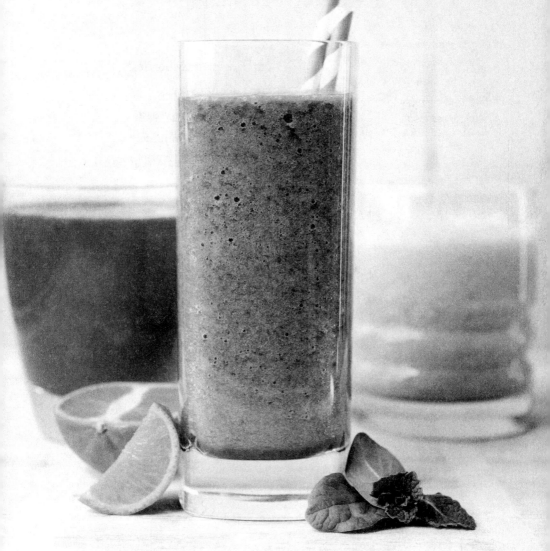

STRAWBERRY COCONUT

*B*right strawberry flavor in a creamy hemp base, this blend has a hint of rosemary and citrus.

Berries contain several phenolic compounds that have the ability to induce apoptosis and suppress cancer genes.

SERVES ❷

1 cup frozen strawberries

1 cup coconut water

¼ cup hulled hemp seed

2 teaspoons lemon juice

½ teaspoon rosemary leaf powder

Combine all ingredients in a high-power blender or food processor and blend until smooth. Drink immediately.

Nutrition Facts *(per serving)*

Calories 140; Fat 9; Protein 7; Carbs 8; Fiber 3; Net Carbs 5

Research Study

R. R. Somasagara, M. Hegde, K. K. Chiruvella, et al. (2012). Extracts of strawberry fruits induce intrinsic pathway of apoptosis in breast cancer cells and inhibits tumor progression in mice. *PLoS One* 7 (10): e47021.

WATERMELON LIME

*L*ush watermelon and tart lime complement each other in this cool and fresh smoothie.

Watermelon contains even more lycopene than tomatoes. This antioxidant carotenoid shows an array of biological effects, including reducing inflammation and interfering with breast cancer cell development.

SERVES ❶

1 cup watermelon

½ cup coconut water

2 tablespoons chia seed

1 tablespoon lime juice

Combine all ingredients in a high-power blender or food processor and blend until smooth. Drink immediately.

Nutrition Facts *(per serving)*

Calories 180; Fat 10; Protein 7; Carbs 23; Fiber 13; Net Carbs 10

Research Study

V. Bhuvaneswari and S. Nagini. (2005). Lycopene: A review of its potential as an anticancer agent. *Current Medicinal Chemistry Anticancer Agents* 5 (6): 627–35.

CREAMY CHAI COCOA

This frosty and spicy smoothie is fragrant with spices and sweet like chocolate milk.

Vanilla beans contain piperonal and vanillin, which are cytotoxic compounds that have been found to inhibit human breast cancer cells in laboratory studies. Black pepper contains piperine, a potent compound that has an antitumor effect against breast cancer cells.

SERVES ❷

1 frozen banana

1 cup coconut water

2 tablespoons protein powder

1 tablespoon dark unsweetened cocoa powder

½ teaspoon vanilla extract

Pinch of ground cinnamon

Pinch of ground cloves

Pinch of fresh ground black pepper

Combine all ingredients in a high-power blender or food processor and blend until smooth. Drink immediately.

Nutrition Facts *(per serving)*

Calories 115; Fat 2; Protein 8; Carbs 18; Fiber 6; Net Carbs 12

Research Studies

K. Lirdprapamongkol, H. Sakurai, N. Kawasaki, et al. (2005). Vanillin suppresses in vitro invasion and in vivo metastasis of mouse breast cancer cells. *European Journal of Pharmaceutical Sciences* 25 (1): 57–65.
S. Sriwiriyajan, A. Tedasen, N. Lailerd, et al. (2016). Anticancer and cancer prevention effects of piperine-free *Piper nigrum* extract on N-nitrosomethylurea-induced mammary tumorigenesis in rats. *Cancer Prevention Research* 9 (1): 74–82.

CHERRY CHIA TEA

This sweet and refreshing combination has earthy undertones from the green tea and a little herbal scent from the turmeric.

Piperine, a major alkaloid in black pepper, has diverse physiological actions, including killing cancer cells, inhibiting proliferation of cancer cells, and reducing angiogenesis.

SERVES **1**

½ cup frozen cherries

½ cup coconut water

½ cup green tea ice cubes

2 tablespoons chia seed

¼ teaspoon fresh ground black pepper

Pinch of turmeric powder

Combine all ingredients in a high-power blender or food processor and blend until smooth. Drink immediately.

Nutrition Facts *(per serving)*

Calories 160; Fat 10; Protein 6; Carbs 16; Fiber 13; Net Carbs 3

Research Study

C. D. Doucette, A. L. Hilchie, R. Liwski, et al. (2012). Piperine, a dietary phytochemical, inhibits angiogenesis. *Journal of Nutritional Biochemistry* 24 (1): 231–39.

BANANA ORANGE WHIP

A creamy blend with bright orange flavor, this combination is simple perfection.

The probiotic *Lactobacillus casei* has been found to stimulate an immune response against breast tumors and decrease tumor growth rate.

SERVES ❷

1 frozen banana

1 cup coconut water

½ cup orange

2 tablespoons protein powder

¼ teaspoon probiotic powder

Combine all ingredients in a high-power blender or food processor and blend until smooth. Drink immediately.

Nutrition Facts *(per serving)*

Calories 130; Fat 2; Protein 8; Carbs 21; Fiber 5; Net Carbs 16

Research Study

F. Aragón, S. Carino, G. Perdigón, et al. (2014). The administration of milk fermented by the probiotic *Lactobacillus casei* CRL 431 exerts an immunomodulatory effect against a breast tumour in a mouse model. *Immunobiology* 219 (6): 457–64.

CHOCOLATE POMEGRANATE

*T*his dark chocolate smoothie with tannic pomegranate flavor has a little citrus edge.

Cocoa contains procyanidin compounds that provide protection from proliferation of breast cancer cells.

SERVES ❷

½ cup frozen pineapple

½ cup green tea ice cubes

3 tablespoons pomegranate juice concentrate

2 tablespoons unsweetened cocoa powder

2 tablespoons hulled hemp seed

Combine all ingredients in a high-power blender or food processor and blend until smooth. Drink immediately.

Nutrition Facts *(per serving)*

Calories 110; Fat 5; Protein 5; Carbs 13; Fiber 3; Net Carbs 10

Research Study

D. Ramljak, L. J. Romanczyk, L. J. Metheny-Barlow, et al. (2005). Pentameric procyanidin from *Theobroma cacao* selectively inhibits growth of human breast cancer cells. *Molecular Cancer Therapeutics* 4 (4): 537–46.

FRESH PAPAYA LIME

*T*his light and fresh combination has a delicate papaya flavor with a bit of lime.

Papaya is rich in lycopene, a carotenoid that reduces breast cancer growth in several ways, which include reducing inflammation and inhibiting cell invasion, angiogenesis, and metastasis, as well as triggering apoptosis.

SERVES ❶

1 cup papaya
½ cup coconut water
2 tablespoons chia seed
1 tablespoon lime juice
Pinch of turmeric powder

Combine all ingredients in a high-power blender or food processor and blend until smooth. Drink immediately.

Nutrition Facts *(per serving)*

Calories 210; Fat 10; Protein 7; Carbs 30; Fiber 15; Net Carbs 15

Research Study

M. Ono, M. Takeshima, and S. Nakano. (2015). Mechanism of the anticancer effect of lycopene (Tetraterpenoids). *Enzymes* 37:139–66.

LUSCIOUS TART CHERRY

*P*eaches mellow the intense cherry flavor in this rich combination.

Tart cherries are rich in anthocyanins that have the ability to reduce breast cancer cells via apoptosis.

SERVES ❶

½ cup frozen tart cherries

½ cup frozen peaches

½ cup coconut water

2 tablespoons chia seed

½ teaspoon probiotic powder

½ teaspoon turmeric powder

Combine all ingredients in a high-power blender or food processor and blend until smooth. Drink immediately.

Nutrition Facts *(per serving)*

Calories 220; Fat 10; Protein 7; Carbs 30; Fiber 15; Net Carbs 15

Research Study

K. R. Martin and A. Wooden. (2012). Tart cherry juice induces differential dose-dependent effects on apoptosis, but not cellular proliferation, in MCF-7 human breast cancer cells. *Journal of Medicinal Food* 15 (11): 945–54.

COCONUT PEACH AND BERRY

*S*weet peaches and strawberries pair well with coconut water in this delicious and light smoothie.

A higher intake of berries and peaches is associated with lower risk of ER- (estrogen receptor negative) breast cancer among postmenopausal women.

SERVES ❷

1 cup coconut water

½ cup frozen peaches

½ cup frozen strawberries

2 tablespoons chia seed

½ teaspoon turmeric powder

Combine all ingredients in a high-power blender or food processor and blend until smooth. Drink immediately.

Nutrition Facts *(per serving)*

Calories 100; Fat 5; Protein 4; Carbs 12; Fiber 7; Net Carbs 5

Research Study

T. T. Fung, S. E. Chiuve, W. C. Willett, et al. (2013). Intake of specific fruits and vegetables in relation to risk of estrogen receptor-negative breast cancer among postmenopausal women. *Breast Cancer Treatment and Research* 138 (3): 925–30.

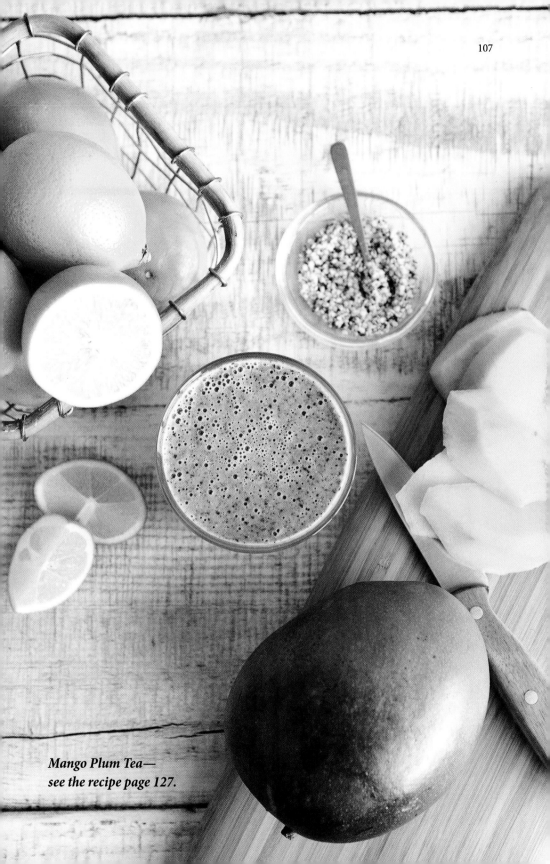

Mango Plum Tea—
see the recipe page 127.

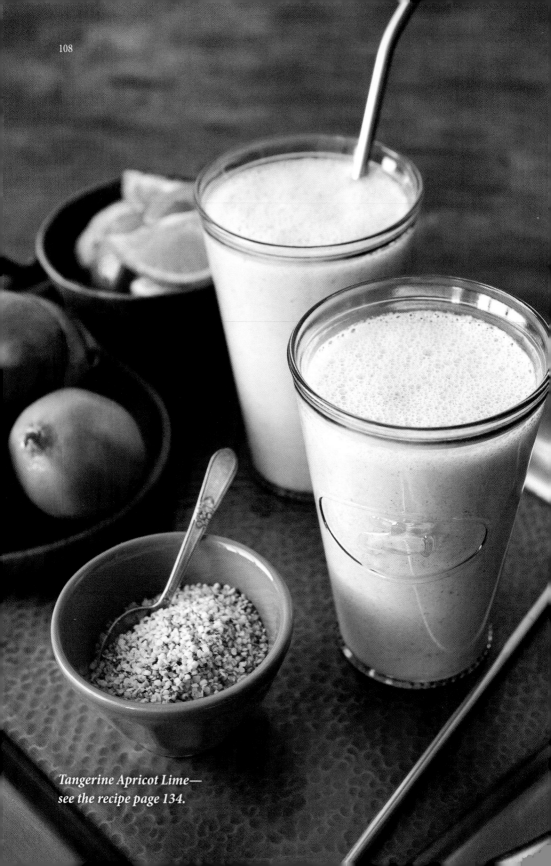

*Tangerine Apricot Lime—
see the recipe page 134.*

*Rosemary Watermelon—
see the recipe page 136.*

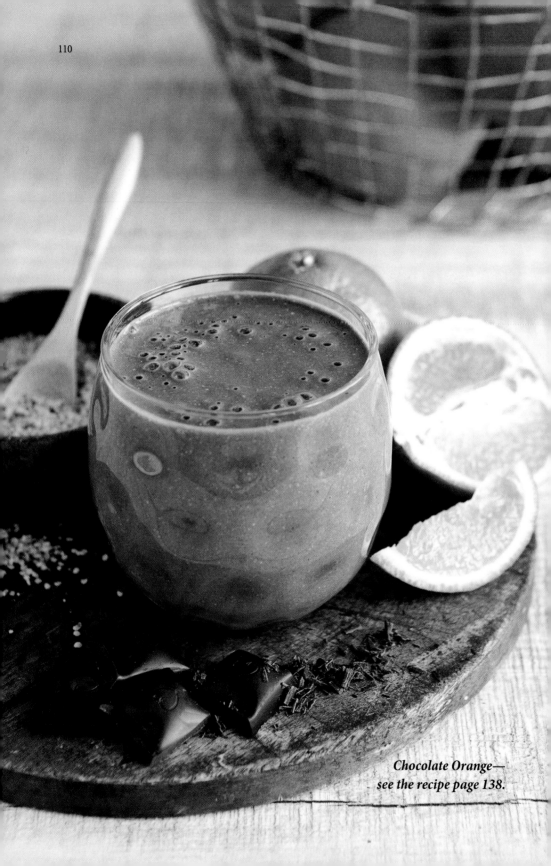

Chocolate Orange—
see the recipe page 138.

ELLAGIC MAGIC

This heavenly smoothie has a creamy texture with intense pink color (see photo page 81) and layers of fresh flavor!

Peaches, grapes, and raspberries are all rich sources of ellagic acid, a cancer-inhibiting phenolic compound. Ellagic acid has been found to reverse cancer cell replication and stimulate apoptosis in estrogen-mediated breast cancer.

SERVES ❷

½ cup frozen peaches

½ cup grapes

½ cup frozen raspberries

½ cup coconut water

¼ cup hulled hemp seed

Combine all ingredients in a high-power blender or food processor and blend until smooth. Drink immediately.

Nutrition Facts *(per serving)*

Calories 150; Fat 9; Protein 7; Carbs 10; Fiber 4; Net Carbs 6

Research Study

R. Munagala, F. Aqil, M. V. Vadhanam, et al. (2013). MicroRNA "signature" during estrogen-mediated mammary carcinogenesis and its reversal by ellagic acid intervention. *Cancer Letters* 339 (2): 175–84.

BASIL LIME

This green tea and basil combination is light and aromatic and tastes a bit like a virgin cocktail.

This refreshing smoothie is low in calories and loaded with nutrients, flavor, and electrolytes. Green tea catechins provide protection against breast cancer by modulating breast cell carcinogenesis.

SERVES ❷

1 cup coconut water

1 cup green tea ice cubes

½ cup fresh basil leaves

2 tablespoons chia seed

1 tablespoon lime juice

Combine all ingredients in a high-power blender or food processor and blend until smooth. Drink immediately.

Nutrition Facts *(per serving)*

Calories 70; Fat 5; Protein 3; Carbs 6; Fiber 6; Net Carbs 0

Research Study

E. C. Yiannakopoulou. (2013). Effect of green tea catechins on breast carcinogenesis: A systematic review of in-vitro and in-vivo experimental studies. *European Journal of Cancer Prevention* 23 (2): 84–89.

WILD BLUEBERRY CHERRY

Intense cherry and wild blueberry flavor is balanced by the green tea cubes in this cool blend.

Inflammation is a major cause of fatigue in cancer survivors. Omega-3 fatty acids, found in chia seed, help reduce this inflammation and its resulting fatigue.

SERVES ❷

1 cup frozen wild blueberries

½ cup frozen cherries

½ cup coconut water

2 tablespoons chia seed

½ teaspoon turmeric powder

Combine all ingredients in a high-power blender or food processor and blend until smooth. Drink immediately.

Nutrition Facts *(per serving)*

Calories 130; Fat 6; Protein 4; Carbs 18; Fiber 8; Net Carbs 10

Research Study

C. M. Alfano, I. Imayama, M. L. Neuhouser, et al. (2012). Fatigue, inflammation, and ω-3 and ω-6 fatty acid intake among breast cancer survivors. *Journal of Clinical Oncology* 30 (12): 1280–87.

COCONUT STRAWBERRY FROSTY

This simple berry and vanilla combination is rich in satisfying protein.

Strawberries contain ellagic acid, an anticancer agent that is being studied as a treatment for breast cancer.

SERVES ❷

1 cup coconut water

1 cup frozen strawberries

2 tablespoons protein powder

2 tablespoons hulled hemp seed

1 vanilla bean

Combine all ingredients in a high-power blender or food processor and blend until smooth. Drink immediately.

Nutrition Facts *(per serving)*

Calories 130; Fat 6; Protein 11; Carbs 10; Fiber 5; Net Carbs 5

Research Study

R. Munagala, F. Aqil, M. V. Vadhanam, et al. (2013). MicroRNA "signature" during estrogen-mediated mammary carcinogenesis and its reversal by ellagic acid intervention. *Cancer Letters* 339 (2): 175–84.

RASPBERRY COCONUT FROSTY

*C*oconut and raspberry flavors really pop in this cool and light blend.

Raspberries contain anthocyanins that provide protection against breast cancer when combined with probiotics, such as those found in cultured coconut milk.

SERVES ❶

½ cup cultured coconut milk

½ cup coconut water

½ cup frozen raspberries

2 tablespoons hulled hemp seed

Combine all ingredients in a high-power blender or food processor and blend until smooth. Drink immediately.

Nutrition Facts *(per serving)*

Calories 240; Fat 17; Protein 10; Carbs 16; Fiber 9; Net Carbs 7

Research Study

T. Tarko, A. Duda-Chodak, and N. Zajac. (2013). Digestion and absorption of phenolic compounds assessed by in vitro simulation methods. *Roczniki Państwowego Zakładu Higieny* 64 (2): 79–84.

GREEN TEA
SMOOTHIES

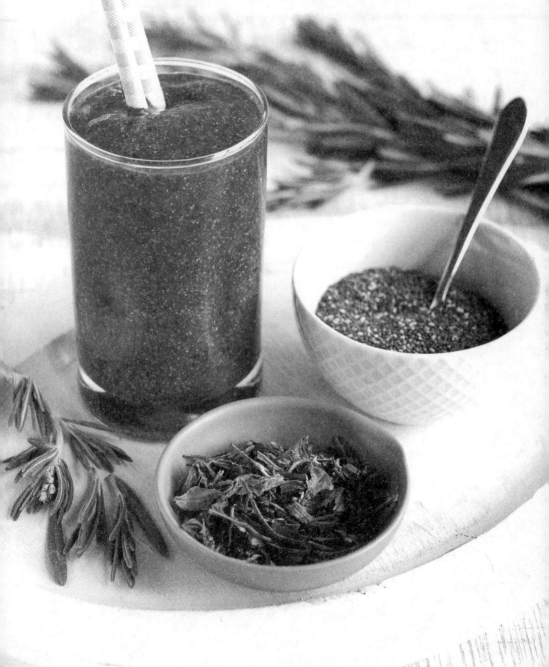

CHERRY MELON LIME

*T*his creamy blend is complex and refreshing, with a fresh cantaloupe base and layers of cherry, green tea, and lime.

Scientists have shown that EGCG suppresses the growth, migration, and invasion of human breast cancer by inhibiting blood flow to the cancer cells.

SERVES ❷

1 cup green tea ice cubes

½ cup cantaloupe

3 tablespoons black cherry juice concentrate

2 tablespoons hulled hemp seed

1 teaspoon lime juice

½ teaspoon rosemary leaf powder

Combine all ingredients in a high-power blender or food processor and blend until smooth. Drink immediately.

Nutrition Facts *(per serving)*

Calories 90; Fat 5; Protein 4; Carbs 9; Fiber 1; Net Carbs 8

Research Study

E. C. Yiannakopoulou. (2013). Effect of green tea catechins on breast carcinogenesis: A systematic review of in-vitro and in-vivo experimental studies. *European Journal of Cancer Prevention* 23 (2): 84–89.

CARDAMOM CHOCOLATE WHIP

Chocolaty sweet, this luscious combination has a strong cardamom flavor and scent.

Limonene is a bioactive food compound found in cardamom pods that concentrates in breast tissues and has preventive and therapeutic effects on breast cancer.

SERVES ❷

1 vanilla bean

1 cup green tea ice cubes

½ cup frozen strawberries

½ cup coconut water

2 tablespoons protein powder

1 tablespoon unsweetened cocoa powder

½ teaspoon cardamom powder

Combine all ingredients in a high-power blender or food processor and blend until smooth. Drink immediately.

Nutrition Facts *(per serving)*

Calories 70; Fat 2; Protein 8; Carbs 8; Fiber 5; Net Carbs 3

Research Study

A. Acharya, I. Das, S. Singh, et al. (2010). Chemopreventive properties of indole-3-carbinol, diindolylmethane and other constituents of cardamom against carcinogenesis. *Recent Patents of Food, Nutrition and Agriculture* 2 (2): 166–77.

STRAWBERRY BASIL CITRUS

*T*his strange and delicious blend has fresh herbal and sweet berry flavors.

Curcumin, an active compound in turmeric, inhibits breast cancer cell growth and induces apoptosis in human breast cancer cells.

SERVES ❷

1 cup green tea ice cubes

½ cup tangerine juice

½ cup frozen strawberries

½ cup fresh basil leaves

2 tablespoons hulled hemp seed

½ teaspoon turmeric powder

Combine all ingredients in a high-power blender or food processor and blend until smooth. Drink immediately.

Nutrition Facts *(per serving)*

Calories 100; Fat 5; Protein 4; Carbs 11; Fiber 2; Net Carbs 9

Research Study

Y. Xia, L. Jin, B. Zhang, et al. (2007). The potentiation of curcumin on insulin-like growth factor-1 action in MCF-7 human breast carcinoma cells. *Life Sciences* 80 (23): 2161–69.

HESPERIDIN TONIC

*T*his citus and berry combination is tangy and sweet.

Tangerines contain the flavonoid hesperidin, an antioxidant compound that inhibits the growth and replication of hormone-sensitive breast cancer cells.

SERVES ❷

1 tangerine

1 cup brewed green tea

1 cup frozen strawberries

2 tablespoons chia seed

Combine all ingredients in a high-power blender or food processor and blend until smooth. Drink immediately.

Nutrition Facts *(per serving)*

Calories 130; Fat 5; Protein 4; Carbs 21; Fiber 9; Net Carbs 12

Research Study

C. J. Lee, L. Wilson, M. A. Jordan, et al. (2009). Hesperidin suppressed proliferations of both human breast cancer and androgen-dependent prostate cancer cells. *Phytotherapy Research* 24 Suppl 1: S15–19.

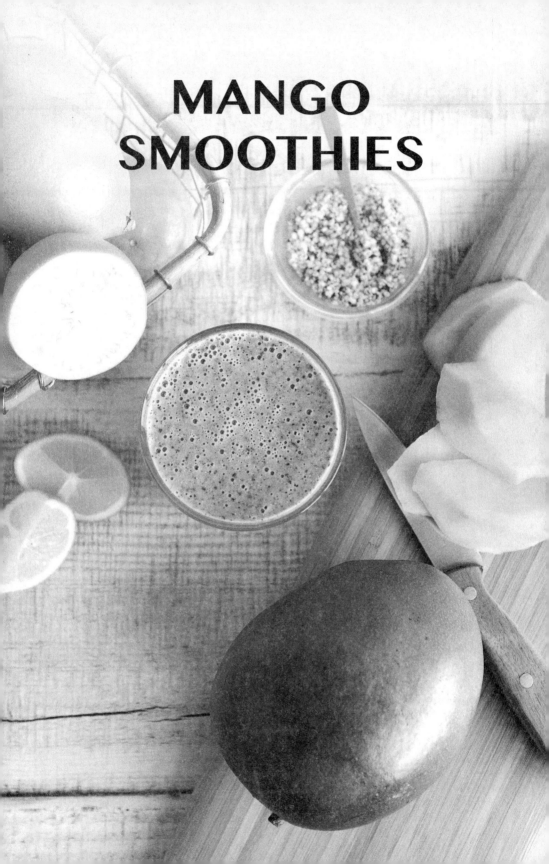

MANGO SMOOTHIES

CREAMY GOLDEN MANGO

*R*ich and creamy, this blend is like a milkshake with exotic mango and turmeric flavors.

Bananas and green tea provide catechins that directly support the healing of breast cancer by anti-angiogenesis, which is the reduction of the blood supply to cancer cells.

SERVES ❷

1 frozen banana

½ cup mango nectar

½ cup green tea cubes

2 tablespoons protein powder

½ teaspoon turmeric powder

Combine all ingredients in a high-power blender or food processor and blend until smooth. Drink immediately.

Nutrition Facts *(per serving)*

Calories 140; Fat 2; Protein 8; Carbs 24; Fiber 5; Net Carbs 19

Research Study

E. C. Yiannakopoulou. (2013). Green tea catechins: Proposed mechanisms of action in breast cancer focusing on the interplay between survival and apoptosis. *Anticancer Agents Medicinal Chemistry* 14 (2): 290–95.

PINK MANGO BERRY

*C*reamy and smooth, this blend has intense, mouthwatering raspberry flavor!

Mangiferin is a bioactive xanthonoid, or a natural plant polyphenol, found in mango that has the ability to reduce cancer cell growth by apoptosis.

SERVES **1**

½ cup mango nectar

½ cup frozen raspberries

2 tablespoons protein powder

½ teaspoon turmeric powder

Combine all ingredients in a high-power blender or food processor and blend until smooth. Drink immediately.

Nutrition Facts *(per serving)*

Calories 170; Fat 3; Protein 14; Carbs 21; Fiber 6; Net Carbs 15

Research Study

Matkowski, P. Kuś́, E. Góralska, et al. (2013). Mangiferin—a bioactive xanthonoid, not only from mango and not just antioxidant. *Mini Reviews in Medicinal Chemistry* 13 (3): 439–55.

GOLDEN BASIL BERRY

*T*his fresh basil smoothie has a subtle green color in a light and
creamy base.

Turmeric and basil contain
bioactive compounds that
help reduce cancer cell
growth.

SERVES ❷

½ cup mango nectar

½ cup frozen strawberries

½ cup green tea ice cubes

½ cup fresh basil leaves

2 tablespoons hulled hemp seed

½ teaspoon turmeric powder

Pinch of fresh ground black pepper

Combine all ingredients in a high-
power blender or food processor and
blend until smooth. Drink immediately.

Nutrition Facts *(per serving)*

Calories 100; Fat 5; Protein 4; Carbs 12; Fiber 2; Net Carbs 10

Research Study

J. Lv, Q. Shao, H. Wang, et al. (2013). Effects and mechanisms of curcumin and basil polysaccharide on the invasion of SKOV3 cells and dendritic cells. *Molecular Medicine Reports* 92 (2): 218–31.

MANGO PLUM TEA

*T*his fresh mango smoothie has a soft pretty color (see photo page 107) with a bit of tart lemon and a sweet plum base.

Plums contain isatin, an indole, found to trigger apoptosis of human breast cancer cells that are estrogen receptor positive.

SERVES ❷

1 plum

½ cup mango nectar

½ cup green tea ice cubes

¼ cup hulled hemp seed

1 teaspoon lemon juice

Combine all ingredients in a high-power blender or food processor and blend until smooth. Drink immediately.

Nutrition Facts *(per serving)*

Calories 160; Fat 9; Protein 7; Carbs 13; Fiber 2; Net Carbs 11

Research Study

A. A. Radwan, F. K. Alanazi, and A. Al-Dhfyan. (2013). Synthesis, and docking studies of some fused-quinazolines and quinazolines carrying biological active isatin moiety as cell-cycle inhibitors of breast cancer cell lines. *Drug Research* 63 (3): 129–36.

RASPBERRY BANANA MANGO

This fresh tropical blend has a sharp raspberry bite and sweet banana flavor.

Raspberries, bananas, and mango contain antioxidants, which appear to inhibit the growth of breast cancer cells.

SERVES ❸

½ frozen banana

1 cup frozen raspberries

½ cup mango nectar

½ cup green tea ice cubes

2 tablespoons chia seed

½ teaspoon turmeric powder

Combine all ingredients in a high-power blender or food processor and blend until smooth. Drink immediately.

Nutrition Facts *(per serving)*

Calories 105; Fat 3; Protein 3; Carbs 19; Fiber 7; Net Carbs 12

Research Study

I. Jordan, A. Hebestreit, B. Swai, et al. (2013). Dietary patterns and breast cancer risk among women in northern Tanzania: A case-control study. *European Journal of Nutrition* 52 (3): 905–15.

SUPER MANGO

*T*his rich smoothie has the flavor and the fragrance of the tropics.

Mango fruit contains polyphenolics, including gallic acid and gallotannins, that are anti-inflammatory and cytotoxic to breast cancer cells.

SERVES ❷

1 cup mango nectar

1 cup green tea ice cubes

½ cup frozen pineapple

¼ cup hulled hemp seed

2 teaspoons lemon juice

Combine all ingredients in a high-power blender or food processor and blend until smooth. Drink immediately.

Nutrition Facts *(per serving)*

Calories 200; Fat 9; Protein 7; Carbs 22; Fiber 2; Net Carbs 20

Research Study

N. Banerjee, H. Kim, K. Krenek, et al. (2015). Mango polyphenolics suppressed tumor growth in breast cancer xenografts in mice: Role of the PI3K/AKT pathway and associated microRNAs. *Nutrition Research* 35 (8): 744–51.

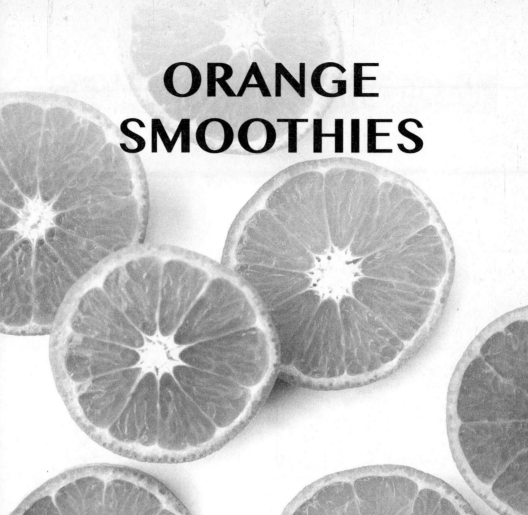

ORANGE
SMOOTHIES

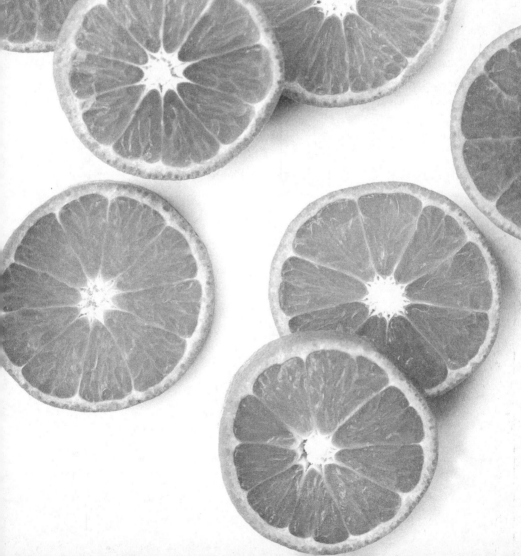

RASPBERRY ORANGE GINGER

*T*his smoothie has sweet berry flavor, bright raspberry color, heat from the ginger, and fresh basil fragrance.

Hesperidin, a flavanone glycoside found in citrus fruits, exhibits a significant cytotoxic effect in human breast carcinoma and is particularly effective in preventing and healing hormone-sensitive cancers.

SERVES ❷

½ cup fresh basil leaves

½ cup orange juice

½ cup green tea ice cubes

½ cup frozen raspberries

2 tablespoons hulled hemp seed

1 teaspoon fresh ginger root

Combine all ingredients in a high-power blender or food processor and blend until smooth. Drink immediately.

Nutrition Facts *(per serving)*

Calories 110; Fat 5; Protein 5; Carbs 13; Fiber 3; Net Carbs 10

Research Study

C. J. Lee, L. Wilson, M. A. Jordan, et al. (2009). Hesperidin suppressed proliferations of both human breast cancer and androgen-dependent prostate cancer cells. *Phytotherapy Research* 24 Suppl 1: S15–19.

CANTALOUPE ORANGE BASIL

*T*his light and fresh melon smoothie is not too sweet and has an herbal fragrance.

Limonene, a bioactive oil found in citrus juices and in citrus peel, reduces breast cancer cell growth in women with early-stage breast cancer.

SERVES ❷

1 cup cantaloupe

½ cup fresh basil leaves

½ cup orange juice

¼ cup hulled hemp seed

1 teaspoon lemon juice

Combine all ingredients in a high-power blender or food processor and blend until smooth. Drink immediately.

Nutrition Facts *(per serving)*

Calories 180; Fat 9; Protein 8; Carbs 17; Fiber 3; Net Carbs 14

Research Study

J. A. Miller, J. E. Lang, M. Ley, et al. (2013). Human breast tissue disposition and bioactivity of limonene in women with early-stage breast cancer. *Cancer Prevention Research* 6 (6): 577–84.

TANGERINE APRICOT LIME

*T*his bright orange smoothie (see photo page 108) has layers of fresh fruit flavor.

Nobiletin is a bioflavonoid found in citrus fruits— such as lemons, oranges, tangerines, and grapefruits—that has the potential to suppress metastasis of breast cancer via its anti-inflammatory and anticancer activities.

SERVES ❷

1 tangerine

1 apricot

½ cup orange juice

½ cup green tea ice cubes

¼ cup hulled hemp seed

1 tablespoon lime juice

Combine all ingredients in a high-power blender or food processor and blend until smooth. Drink immediately.

Nutrition Facts *(per serving)*

Calories 180; Fat 9; Protein 8; Carbs 19; Fiber 3; Net Carbs 16

Research Study

S. H. Baek, S. M. Kim, D. Nam, et al. (2012). Antimetastatic effect of nobiletin through the down-regulation of CXC chemokine receptor type 4 and matrix metallopeptidase-9. *Pharmaceutical Biology* 50 (10): 1210–18.

ORANGE CRANBERRY BASIL

This smoothie is exotic with intense berry flavor and has the perfect blend of cranberry and basil.

Cranberry juice is an abundant source of flavonoids, such as quercetin, proanthocyanidins, and flavonols. Quercetin supports breast cancer recovery by inhibiting cancer cell growth and inducing apoptosis.

SERVES ❷

½ cup orange juice

½ cup cranberry juice

½ cup frozen wild blueberries

½ cup fresh basil leaves

2 tablespoons protein powder

2 tablespoons hulled hemp seed

Combine all ingredients in a high-power blender or food processor and blend until smooth. Drink immediately.

Nutrition Facts *(per serving)*

Calories 170; Fat 6; Protein 11; Carbs 18; Fiber 5; Net Carbs 13

Research Study

J. Duo, G. G. Ying, G. W. Wang, et al. (2012). Quercetin inhibits human breast cancer cell proliferation and induces apoptosis via Bcl-2 and Bax regulation. *Molecular Medicine Reports* 5 (6): 1453–56.

ROSEMARY WATERMELON

*T*his bright pink smoothie (see photo page 109) has complex fruit flavors with light rosemary fragrance.

Naringin, a major flavonoid in citrus fruits, inhibits the growth of triple-negative (ER-/PR-/HER2-) breast cancer.

SERVES ❷

1 cup orange juice

1 cup watermelon

½ cup frozen strawberries

¼ cup hulled hemp seed

2 teaspoons lime juice

½ teaspoon turmeric powder

½ teaspoon rosemary leaf powder

Pinch of fresh ground black pepper

Combine all ingredients in a high-power blender or food processor and blend until smooth. Drink immediately.

Nutrition Facts *(per serving)*

Calories 180; Fat 9; Protein 8; Carbs 18; Fiber 3; Net Carbs 15

Research Study

H. Li, B. Yang, J. Huang, et al. (2013). Naringin inhibits growth potential of human triple-negative breast cancer cells by targeting β-catenin signaling pathway. *Toxicology Letters* 220 (3): 219–28.

RASPBERRY CITRUS TEA

*T*his citrus smoothie has rich raspberry flavor and just a bit of tartness.

Nutrients in citrus fruits and in citrus peel have the ability to reduce the number of breast cancer cells and enhance some chemotherapeutic agents.

SERVES **2**

½ cup frozen raspberries

½ cup orange juice

½ cup grapefruit juice

½ cup green tea ice cubes

2 tablespoons chia seed

Combine all ingredients in a high-power blender or food processor and blend until smooth. Drink immediately.

Nutrition Facts *(per serving)*

Calories 150; Fat 5; Protein 4; Carbs 25; Fiber 9; Net Carbs 16

Research Study

A. B. Adina, F. A. Goenadi, F. F. Handoko, et al. (2014). Combination of ethanolic extract of Citrus aurantifolia peels with doxorubicin modulate cell cycle and increase apoptosis induction on MCF-7 cells. *Iranian Journal of Pharmaceutical Research* 13 (3): 919–26.

CHOCOLATE ORANGE

*T*his dessert-like treat is sweet, rich, and satisfying, with bold, dark chocolate flavor. See photo page 110.

Hesperidin, a flavonoid found abundantly in oranges and orange juice, has been found to block the growth of breast cancer cells in laboratory studies.

SERVES ❷

1 orange

½ cup orange juice

½ cup green tea ice cubes

2 tablespoons hulled hemp seed

2 tablespoons unsweetened cocoa powder

2 tablespoons protein powder

Combine all ingredients in a high-power blender or food processor and blend until smooth. Drink immediately.

Nutrition Facts *(per serving)*

Calories 180; Fat 7; Protein 12; Carbs 21; Fiber 7; Net Carbs 14

Research Study

T. Tanaka, T. Tanaka, M. Tanaka, et al. (2011). Cancer chemoprevention by citrus pulp and juices containing high amounts of β-cryptoxanthin and hesperidin. *BioMed Research International* 2012:516981.

ORANGE PLUM ROSEMARY

*B*right fruit flavors and lemony tartness are just bursting from this creamy orange smoothie.

Rosemary's carnosic and rosmarinic acid inhibit proliferation of breast cancer cells. Studies have also found that they are particularly effective against estrogen receptor negative (ER-) human breast cancer cells.

SERVES ❷

1 plum

½ cup orange juice

½ cup green tea ice cubes

2 tablespoons hulled hemp seed

¼ teaspoon rosemary leaf powder

2 teaspoons lemon juice

Combine all ingredients in a high-power blender or food processor and blend until smooth. Drink immediately.

Nutrition Facts *(per serving)*

Calories 150; Fat 3; Protein 4; Carbs 24; Fiber 4; Net Carbs 20

Research Study

O. Yesil-Celiktas, C. Sevimli, E. Bedir, et al. (2010). Inhibitory effects of rosemary extracts, carnosic acid and rosmarinic acid on the growth of various human cancer cell lines. *Plant Foods and Human Nutrition* 65 (2): 158–63.

GOLDEN ORANGE PLUM

*O*range and plum flavors sweeten the green tea in this frosty pick-me-up.

Green tea catechins directly target both tumor cells and the blood vessels that feed tumors, thereby inhibiting tumor growth, proliferation, and migration.

SERVES **2**

1 orange

1 plum

½ cup green tea ice cubes

¼ cup hulled hemp seed

½ teaspoon turmeric powder

Combine all ingredients in a high-power blender or food processor and blend until smooth. Drink immediately.

Nutrition Facts *(per serving)*

Calories 150; Fat 5; Protein 4; Carbs 24; Fiber 5; Net Carbs 19

Research Study

J. W. Gu, K. L. Makey, K. B. Tucker, et al. (2013). EGCG, a major green tea catechin suppresses breast tumor angiogenesis and growth via inhibiting the activation of HIF-1α and NFκB, and VEGF expression. *Vascular Cell* 5 (1): 9.

PEACH SMOOTHIES

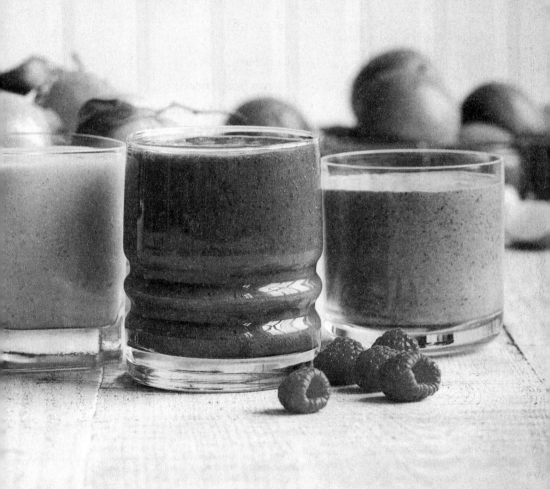

PEACH BASIL SMOOTHIE

*T*his carotene and protein-rich blend has fresh basil fragrance and sweet stone-fruit flavor.

Polyphenolics in peaches and plums reduce breast cancer cells while not affecting normal cells.

SERVES ❷

1 apricot

1 cup peach nectar

½ cup fresh basil leaves

¼ cup hulled hemp seed

½ teaspoon turmeric powder

Combine all ingredients in a high-power blender or food processor and blend until smooth. Drink immediately.

Nutrition Facts *(per serving)*

Calories 190; Fat 9; Protein 7; Carbs 20; Fiber 2; Net Carbs 18

Research Study

M. Vizzotto, W. Porter, D. Byrne, et al. (2014). Polyphenols of selected peach and plum genotypes reduce cell viability and inhibit proliferation of breast cancer cells while not affecting normal cells. *Food Chemistry* 164:363–70.

STRAWBERRY PEACH NECTAR

This blend is rich in polyphenolics and sweet, frosty, rich berry flavor!

Researchers have found that tumor growth and metastasis are inhibited by the intake of two to three peaches per day.

SERVES ❷

2 peaches

½ cup frozen strawberries

½ cup peach nectar

2 tablespoons chia seed

½ teaspoon turmeric powder

Combine all ingredients in a high-power blender or food processor and blend until smooth. Drink immediately.

Nutrition Facts *(per serving)*

Calories 167; Fat 5; Protein 4; Carbs 25; Fiber 9; Net Carbs 16

Research Study

G. Noratto, W. Porter, D. Byrne, et al. (2014). Polyphenolics from peach (*Prunus persica* var. Rich Lady) inhibit tumor growth and metastasis of MDA-MB-435 breast cancer cells in vivo. *Journal of Nutritional Biochemistry* 25 (7): 796–800.

CAROTENOID CRUSH

*T*his sweet and fruity blend is surprisingly citrusy.

The peach nectar, strawberries, and cantaloupe in this smoothie provide alpha- and beta-carotenes. These carotenoids act as cancer-preventive agents by reducing oxidative stress and free radicals in the body.

SERVES ❷

½ cup peach nectar

½ cup frozen strawberries

½ cup cantaloupe

½ cup green tea ice cubes

2 tablespoons chia seed

2 teaspoons lime juice

Combine all ingredients in a high-power blender or food processor and blend until smooth. Drink immediately.

Nutrition Facts *(per serving)*

Calories 130; Fat 5; Protein 4; Carbs 22; Fiber 7; Net Carbs 15

Research Study

A. H. Eliassen, S. J. Hendrickson, L. A. Brinton, et al. (2012). Circulating carotenoids and risk of breast cancer: Pooled analysis of eight prospective studies. *Journal of the National Cancer Institute* 104 (24): 1905–16.

WATERMELON PEACH

*T*his delectable melon and berry blend has a light rosemary accent.

Lycopene, a natural carotenoid, reduces risk for breast cancer development and recurrence. Watermelon is a rich source of lycopene, as it contains about 15 milligrams (mg) in just one slice.

SERVES ❷

½ cup watermelon

½ cup peach nectar

½ cup frozen wild blueberries

2 tablespoons chia seed

½ teaspoon rosemary leaf powder

Combine all ingredients in a high-power blender or food processor and blend until smooth. Drink immediately.

Nutrition Facts *(per serving)*

Calories 140; Fat 5; Protein 4; Carbs 21; Fiber 7; Net Carbs 14

Research Study

R. M. Tamimi, G. A. Colditz, and S. E. Hankinson. (2009). Circulating carotenoids, mammographic density, and subsequent risk of breast cancer. *Cancer Prevention Research* 69 (24): 9323–29.

PINEAPPLE PEACH TEA

*T*his rich and satisfying blend has a light rosemary flavor in a creamy, sweet pineapple base.

Fresh and dried rosemary provide fragrance and flavor and are both rich sources of antioxidants such as rosmarinic acid, which has shown potent action against breast cancer cells.

SERVES **2**

½ cup frozen pineapple

½ cup frozen peaches

½ cup peach nectar

½ cup green tea ice cubes

¼ cup hulled hemp seed

¼ teaspoon rosemary leaf powder

Combine all ingredients in a high-power blender or food processor and blend until smooth. Drink immediately.

Nutrition Facts *(per serving)*

Calories 180; Fat 9; Protein 7; Carbs 14; Fiber 2; Net Carbs 12

Research Study

I. Berdowska, B. Zieliński, I. Fecka, et al. (2013). Cytotoxic impact of phenolics from Lamiaceae species on human breast cancer cells. *Food Chemistry* 41 (2): 1313–21.

CHERRY PEACH TEA

*T*his frosty combination is sweet and aromatic.

Rosemary contains carnosol, an anticancer compound that reduces inflammation and triggers apoptosis of breast cancer cells.

SERVES ❷

½ cup frozen cherries

½ cup peach nectar

½ cup green tea ice cubes

¼ cup hulled hemp seed

½ teaspoon rosemary leaf powder

2 teaspoons lime juice

Combine all ingredients in a high-power blender or food processor and blend until smooth. Drink immediately.

Nutrition Facts *(per serving)*

Calories 170; Fat 8; Protein 7; Carbs 17; Fiber 1; Net Carbs 16

Research Study

J. J. Johnson. (2011). Carnosol: A promising anticancer and anti-inflammatory agent. *Cancer Letters* 305 (1): 1–7.

CRANBERRY PEACH ROSEMARY

The intense herbal flavor is addictive in this rich, tart cranberry base with a slightly sweet peach finish.

Peaches contain ellagic acid, which is a natural compound that provides protection against breast cancer as it turns off genes that are programmed for breast cancer.

SERVES ❶

½ cup frozen peaches

3 tablespoons cranberry juice concentrate

2 tablespoons hulled hemp seed

½ teaspoon rosemary leaf powder

Combine all ingredients in a high-power blender or food processor and blend until smooth. Drink immediately.

Nutrition Facts *(per serving)*

Calories 150; Fat 9; Protein 7; Carbs 12; Fiber 3; Net Carbs 9

Research Study

R. Munagala, F. Aqil, M. V. Vadhanam, et al. (2013). MicroRNA "signature" during estrogen-mediated mammary carcinogenesis and its reversal by ellagic acid intervention. *Cancer Letters* 339 (2): 175–84.

COCONUT MANGO PEACH

*T*his creamy combination has a mellow, soothing flavor and loads of protein.

Mango fruit contains quercetin and norathyriol, which have both been proven to inhibit human breast cancer development.

SERVES ❷

½ cup coconut milk

½ cup frozen mango

½ cup mango nectar

½ cup frozen peaches

¼ cup hulled hemp seed

Combine all ingredients in a high-power blender or food processor and blend until smooth. Drink immediately.

Nutrition Facts *(per serving)*

Calories 220; Fat 12; Protein 8; Carbs 22; Fiber 2; Net Carbs 20

Research Study

A. S. Wilkinson, M. W. Taing, J. T. Pierson, et al. (2015). Estrogen modulation properties of mangiferin and quercetin and the mangiferin metabolite norathyriol. *Food Function* 6 (6): 1847–54.

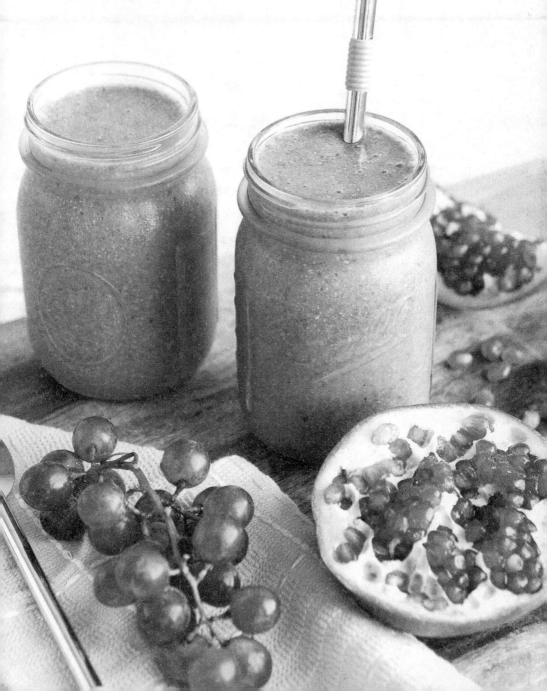

POMEGRANATE
SMOOTHIES

POMEGRANATE GRAPE

Sweet grapes balance the tart pomegranate juice in this protein-rich blend. See photo page 159.

Pomegranate fruit is a source of biologically active compounds with a protective effect against human breast cancer cells.

SERVES ❷

1 cup green tea ice cubes

1 cup frozen grapes

3 tablespoons pomegranate juice concentrate

2 tablespoons chia seed

2 tablespoons protein powder

Combine all ingredients in a high-power blender or food processor and blend until smooth. Drink immediately.

Nutrition Facts *(per serving)*

Calories 190; Fat 7; Protein 11; Carbs 27; Fiber 10; Net Carbs 17

Research Study

S. Sreekumar, H. Sithul, P. Muraleedharan, et al. (2014). Pomegranate fruit as a rich source of biologically active compounds. *BioMed Research International*, article ID 686921.

STRAWBERRY POMEGRANATE

*F*resh strawberries provide a little sweetness to balance the tart pomegranate in this juicy smoothie.

Pomegranate juice contains polyphenols, which have been shown to prevent and reduce the growth of breast cancer cells.

SERVES ❸

1 cup frozen strawberries

½ cup orange juice

3 tablespoons pomegranate juice concentrate

2 tablespoons chia seed

2 tablespoons protein powder

Combine all ingredients in a high-power blender or food processor and blend until smooth. Drink immediately.

Nutrition Facts *(per serving)*

Calories 210; Fat 10; Protein 7; Carbs 29; Fiber 14; Net Carbs 15

Research Study

N. D. Kim, R. Mehta, W. Yu, et al. (2002). Chemopreventive and adjuvant therapeutic potential of pomegranate (*Punica granatum*) for human breast cancer. *Breast Cancer Treatment and Research* 71 (3): 203–17.

POM ORANGE

*S*weet orange juice balances perfectly with the green tea and tannic pomegranate in this smoothie.

Pomegranate seeds contain nutrients that inhibit breast tumors by intervening at various stages of cancer development, including proliferation, invasion, migration, metastasis, angiogenesis, and inflammation.

SERVES ❷

1 orange

1 cup green tea ice cubes

3 tablespoons pomegranate juice concentrate

2 tablespoons chia seed

½ teaspoon turmeric powder

Combine all ingredients in a high-power blender or food processor and blend until smooth. Drink immediately.

Nutrition Facts *(per serving)*

Calories 120; Fat 5; Protein 4; Carbs 20; Fiber 10; Net Carbs 10

Research Study

R. Vini and S. Sreeja. (2015). *Punica granatum* and its therapeutic implications on breast carcinogenesis: A review. *Biofactors* 41 (2): 78–89.

VANILLA PINEAPPLE POMEGRANATE

*T*his blend is creamy, sweet, and frosty, complete with an amazing vanilla and pineapple aroma.

Polyphenols in pomegranate juice reduce breast cancer development by inhibiting its growth and decreasing inflammation.

SERVES **1**

1 vanilla bean

½ cup frozen pineapple

3 tablespoons pomegranate juice concentrate

2 tablespoons protein powder

½ teaspoon turmeric powder

Combine all ingredients in a high-power blender or food processor and blend until smooth. Drink immediately.

Nutrition Facts *(per serving)*

Calories 180; Fat 3; Protein 15; Carbs 26; Fiber 7; Net Carbs 19

Research Study

A. Rocha, L. Wang, M. Penichet, et al. (2012). Pomegranate juice and specific components inhibit cell and molecular processes critical for metastasis of breast cancer. *Breast Cancer Treatment and Research* 136 (3): 647–58.

GREEN TEA POMEGRANATE PINEAPPLE

*T*angy and tart pineapple flavor and tropical sweetness make this smoothie a real treat.

Pineapple contains bromelain, which is a proteolytic enzyme reported to promote apoptosis, particularly in breast cancer cells.

SERVES ❷

1 cup green tea ice cubes

½ cup frozen pineapple

3 tablespoons pomegranate juice concentrate

2 tablespoons chia seed

½ teaspoon rosemary leaf powder

Combine all ingredients in a high-power blender or food processor and blend until smooth. Drink immediately.

Nutrition Facts *(per serving)*

Calories 110; Fat 5; Protein 3; Carbs 15; Fiber 7; Net Carbs 8

Research Study

S. Dhandayuthapani, H. D. Perez, A. Paroulek, et al. (2012). Bromelain-induced apoptosis in GI-101A breast cancer cells. *Journal of Medicinal Food* 15 (4): 344–49.

BLACKBERRY POMEGRANATE

*T*his deep red smoothie has intense blackberry, rosemary, and pomegranate flavors.

Blackberries contain ellagic acid, which is a naturally occurring phytochemical that reduces inflammation, acts as an antioxidant, and triggers apoptosis, destroying breast cancer cells.

SERVES ❷

1 cup green tea ice cubes

1 cup frozen blackberries

3 tablespoons pomegranate juice concentrate

2 tablespoons chia seed

½ teaspoon rosemary leaf powder

Combine all ingredients in a high-power blender or food processor and blend until smooth. Drink immediately.

Nutrition Facts *(per serving)*

Calories 120; Fat 5; Protein 4; Carbs 20; Fiber 10; Net Carbs 10

Research Study

N. P. Seeram, L. S. Adams, Y. Zhang, et al. (2006). Blackberry, black raspberry, blueberry, cranberry, red raspberry, and strawberry extracts inhibit growth and stimulate apoptosis of human cancer cells in vitro. *Journal of Agricultural and Food Chemistry* 54 (25): 9329–39.

KUMQUAT POMEGRANATE CHIA

*T*his smoothie has a deep purple color (see photo page 160). Rich with a wild blueberry and orange wild blueberry, and orange flavor—and an invigorating rosemary fragrance.

Wild blueberries contain concentrated amounts of the antioxidants found in common cultivated berries. For example, Alaskan wild berries ranged from three to five times higher in oxygen radical absorption capacity (ORAC) value when compared to cultivated berries from the lower forty-eight states.

SERVES ❷

6 kumquats

½ cup frozen wild blueberries

3 tablespoons pomegranate juice concentrate

2 tablespoons chia seed

½ teaspoon rosemary leaf powder

Combine all ingredients in a high-power blender or food processor and blend until smooth. Drink immediately.

Nutrition Facts *(per serving)*

Calories 150; Fat 6; Protein 5; Carbs 23; Fiber 11; Net Carbs 12

Research Study

R. R. Dinstel, J. Cascio, and S. Koukel. (2013). The antioxidant level of Alaska's wild berries: High, higher and highest. *International Journal of Circumpolar Health* (August 5): 72.

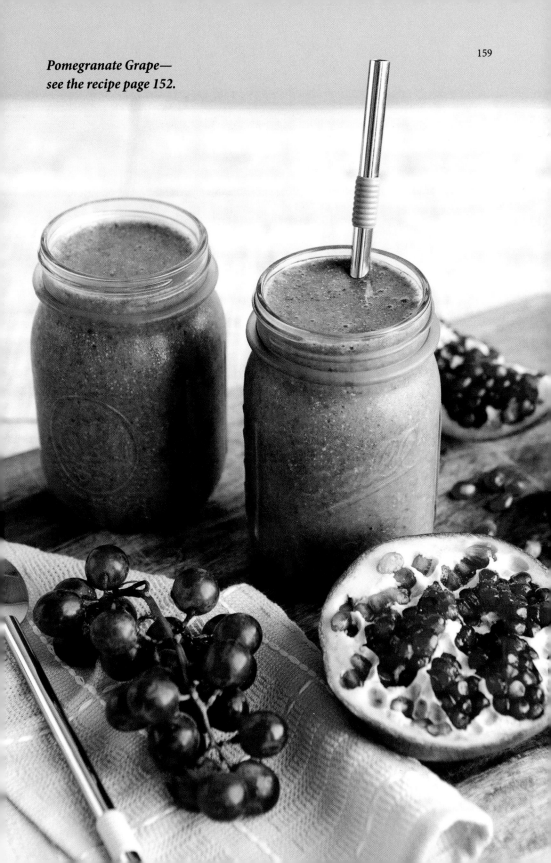

Pomegranate Grape—
see the recipe page 152.

Kumquat Pomegranate Chia—see the recipe page 158.

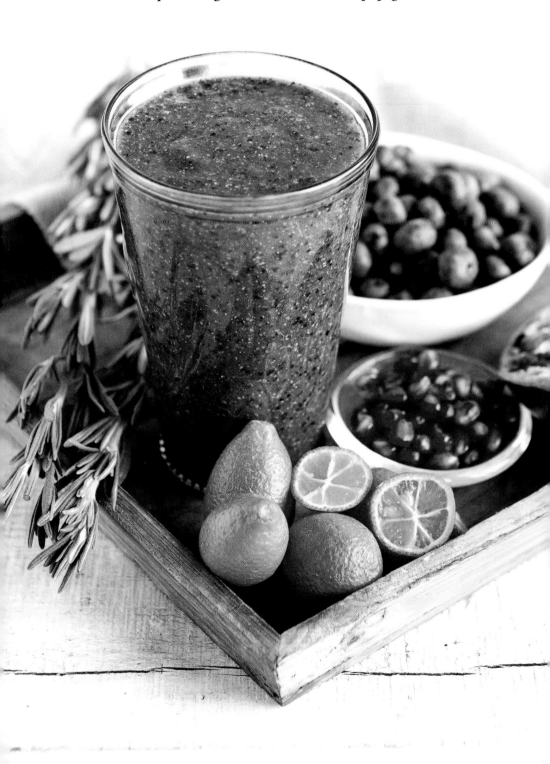

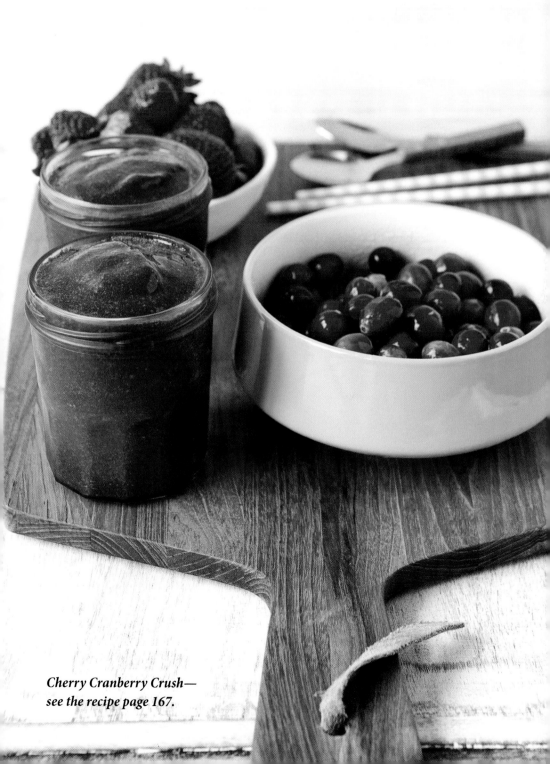

Cherry Cranberry Crush—
see the recipe page 167.

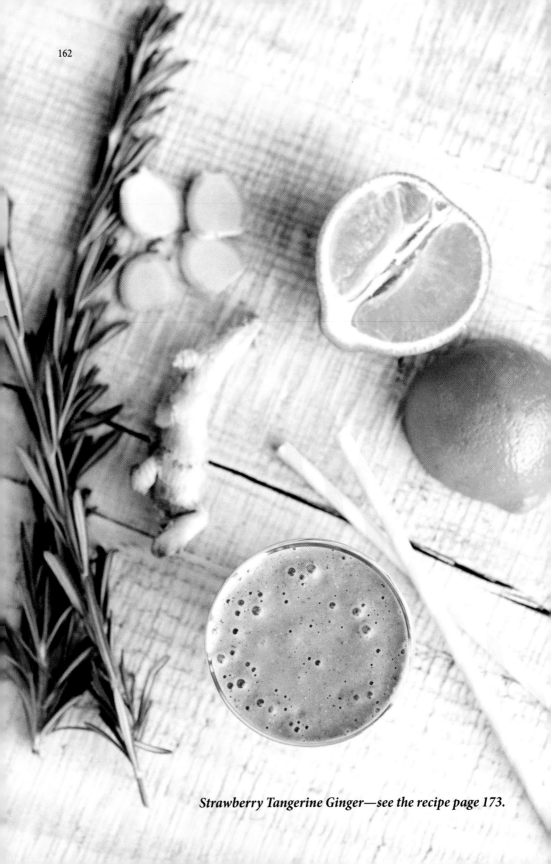

Strawberry Tangerine Ginger—see the recipe page 173.

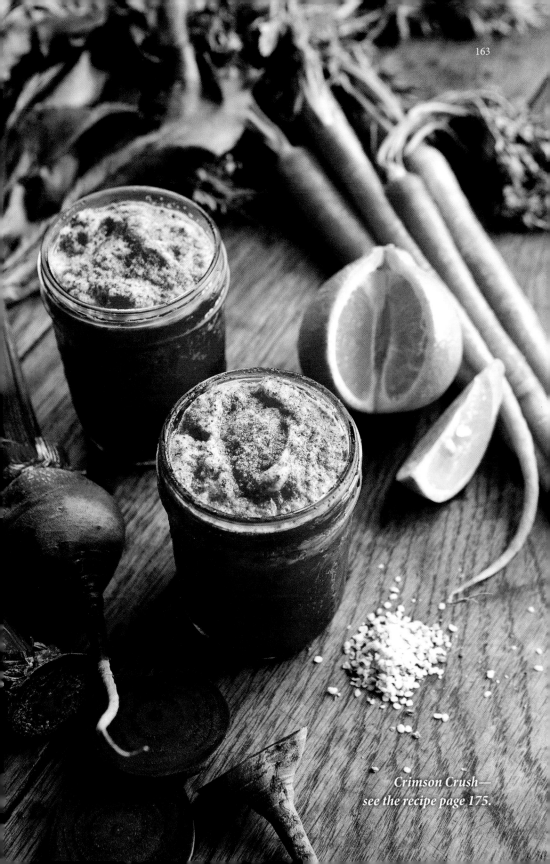

Crimson Crush—
see the recipe page 175.

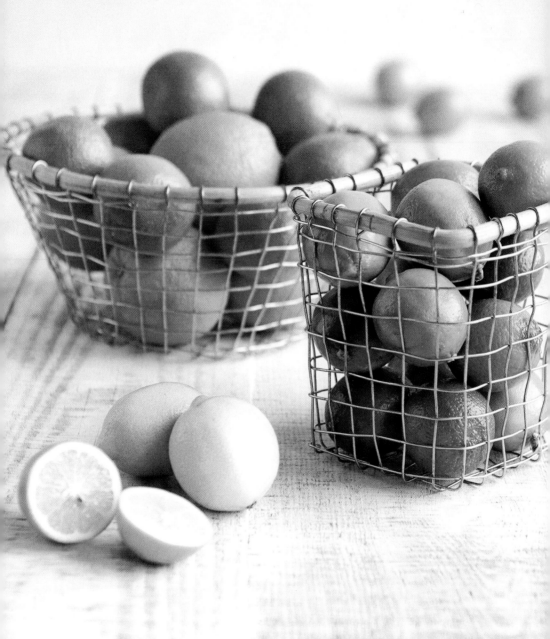

Citrus fruit and citrus peel are rich sources of cancer-inhibiting nutrients, pectin, and oils.

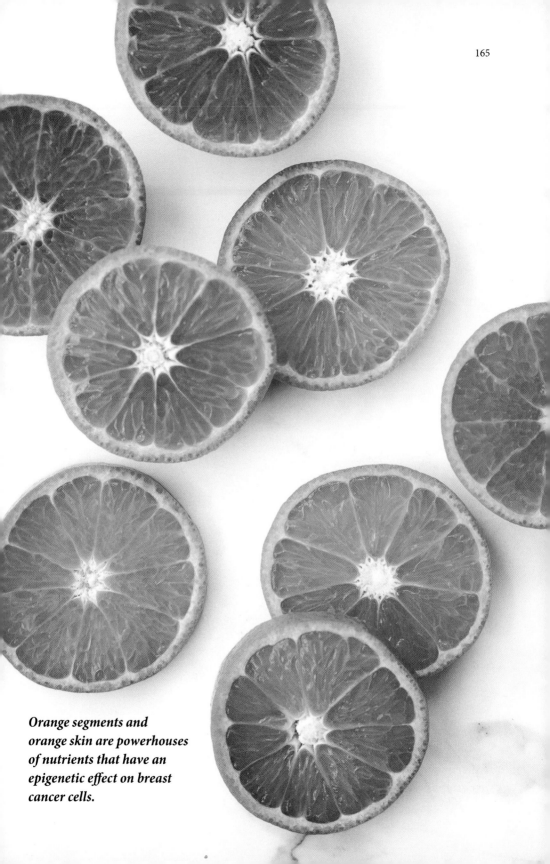

Orange segments and orange skin are powerhouses of nutrients that have an epigenetic effect on breast cancer cells.

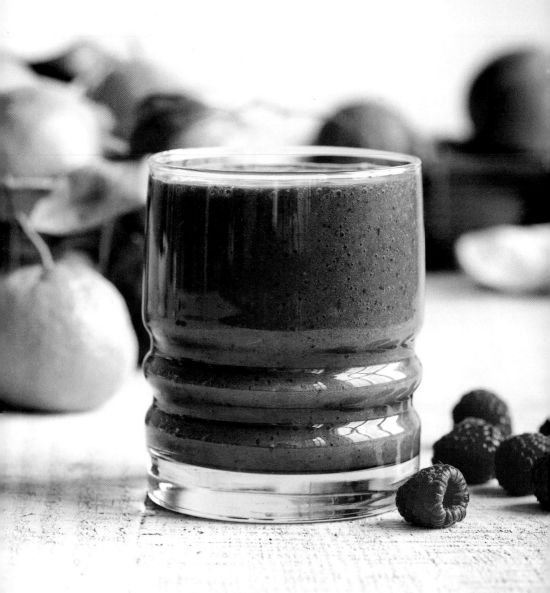

Experiment with a variety of different fruits to customize a smoothie to your taste.

CHERRY CRANBERRY CRUSH

*T*his tasty combination has bright cranberry flavor with a tart finish. See photo page 161.

Cranberries and cranberry juice are rich sources of the antioxidant quercetin, which inhibits breast cancer cell growth and induces apoptosis in human breast cancer cells.

SERVES ❷

½ cup frozen cherries

½ cup coconut water

½ cup green tea ice cubes

¼ cup hulled hemp seed

3 tablespoons cranberry juice concentrate

Combine all ingredients in a high-power blender or food processor and blend until smooth. Drink immediately.

Nutrition Facts *(per serving)*

Calories 140; Fat 9; Protein 7; Carbs 9; Fiber 2; Net Carbs 7

Research Study

J. Duo, G. G. Ying, G. W. Wang, et al. (2012). Quercetin inhibits human breast cancer cell proliferation and induces apoptosis via Bcl-2 and Bax regulation. *Molecular Medicine Reports* 5 (6): 1453–56.

POMEGRANATE ROSEMARY

*F*rosty, thick, and rich, with layers of flavor, this delicious combination is a nutrient powerhouse.

Cherries contain vitamin C and anthocyanins that work together to help reduce the growth of breast cancer cells.

SERVES ❷

½ cup frozen cherries

½ cup green tea ice cubes

3 tablespoons pomegranate juice concentrate

2 tablespoons hulled hemp seed

2 teaspoons lime juice

½ teaspoon rosemary leaf powder

Combine all ingredients in a high-power blender or food processor and blend until smooth. Drink immediately.

Nutrition Facts *(per serving)*

Calories 90; Fat 5; Protein 4; Carbs 10; Fiber 2; Net Carbs 8

Research Study

M. E. Olsson, K. E. Gustavsson, S. Andersson, et al. (2004). Inhibition of cancer cell proliferation in vitro by fruit and berry extracts and correlations with antioxidant levels. *Journal of Agricultural and Food Chemistry* 52 (24): 7264–71.

POMEGRANATE BASIL BERRY

*T*his fruity, herbal blend is heaven in a glass!

Strawberries contain anthocyanins that have an antiproliferative effect on breast cancer cells. Basil contains antioxidants that can reduce cellular damage caused by oxidative stress.

SERVES ❷

½ cup fresh basil leaves

½ cup cantaloupe

½ cup frozen strawberries

¼ cup hulled hemp seed

3 tablespoons pomegranate juice concentrate

Combine all ingredients in a high-power blender or food processor and blend until smooth. Drink immediately.

Nutrition Facts *(per serving)*

Calories 160; Fat 9; Protein 8; Carbs 13; Fiber 3; Net Carbs 10

Research Study

J. Weaver, T. Briscoe, M. Hou, et al. (2009). Strawberry polyphenols are equally cytotoxic to tumorigenic and normal human breast and prostate cell lines. *International Journal of Oncology* 34 (3): 777–86.

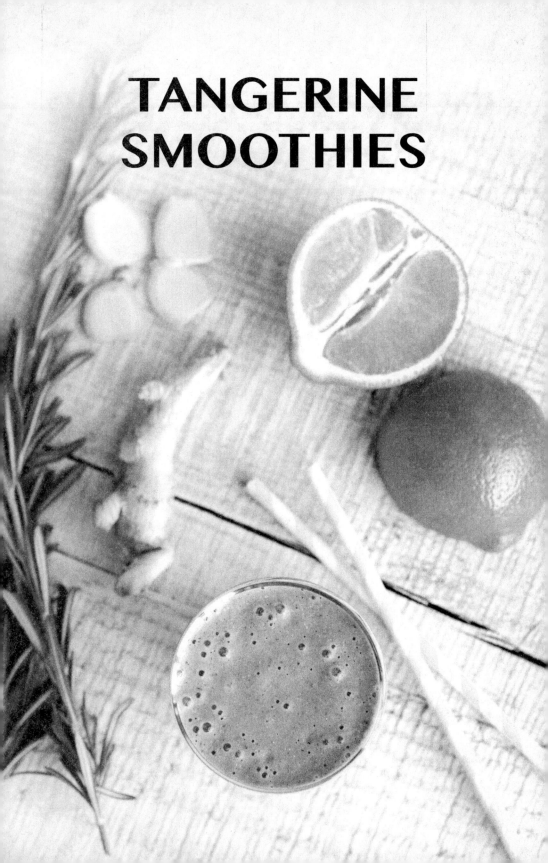

TANGERINE SMOOTHIES

ALPHA CAROTENE TANGERINE

*A*pricot and tangerine flavors mingle perfectly in this tasty combination.

Out of all the carotenoids measured, alpha-carotene, found in apricots and tangerines, was the most predictive of lower levels of cellular oxidation. High cellular oxidation is a biological precursor to many cancers.

SERVES ❷

1 apricot

½ cup tangerine juice

½ cup apricot nectar

½ cup ice

¼ cup hulled hemp seed

Pinch of turmeric

Combine all ingredients in a high-power blender or food processor and blend until smooth. Drink immediately.

Nutrition Facts *(per serving)*

Calories 130; Fat 5; Protein 2; Carbs 17; Fiber 1; Net Carbs 16

Research Study

A. H. Eliassen, S. J. Hendrickson, L. A. Brinton, et al. (2012). Circulating carotenoids and risk of breast cancer: Pooled analysis of eight prospective studies. *Journal of the National Cancer Institute* 104 (24): 1905–16.

STRAWBERRY TANGERINE GINGER

*T*his bright bubble gum-pink smoothie has cool berry flavor with a little heat from the ginger. See photo page 162.

Citrus flavonoids, such as tangeretin, nobiletin, hesperetin, hesperidin, naringenin, and naringin, exert anticancer effects, such as inhibiting cell proliferation and promoting cancer cell apoptosis.

SERVES ❷

1 tangerine

1 cup frozen strawberries

1 cup green tea

2 tablespoons protein powder

1 teaspoon fresh ginger root

¼ teaspoon rosemary leaf powder

Combine all ingredients in a high-power blender or food processor and blend until smooth. Drink immediately.

Nutrition Facts *(per serving)*

Calories 110; Fat 2; Protein 8; Carbs 18; Fiber 6; Net Carbs 12

Research Study

E. Meiyanto, A. Hermawan, and Anindyajati. (2012). Natural products for cancer-targeted therapy: Citrus flavonoids as potent chemopreventive agents. *Asian Pacific Journal of Cancer Prevention* 13 (2): 427–36.

TANGERINE DREAM

*G*orgeous bright pink color—this smoothie is rich in sweet strawberry and
tart cranberry flavors.

Citrus, such as oranges,
tangerines, and grapefruit,
are rich in nobiletin,
which has the potential
to suppress metastasis of
breast cancer.

SERVES ❷

1 cup frozen strawberries

½ cup tangerine juice

3 tablespoons cranberry juice
   concentrate

¼ cup hulled hemp seed

Combine all ingredients in a high-
power blender or food processor and
blend until smooth. Drink immediately.

Nutrition Facts *(per serving)*

Calories 110; Fat 5; Protein 4; Carbs 15; Fiber 2; Net Carbs 13

Research Study

S. H. Baek, S. M. Kim, D. Nam, et al. (2012). Antimetastatic effect of nobiletin through the down-regulation of CXC chemokine
receptor type 4 and matrix metallopeptidase-9. *Pharmaceutical Biology* 50 (10): 1210–18.

CRIMSON CRUSH

*T*his rich smoothie has bright crimson color (see photo page 163) and fresh citrus and carrot juice flavors.

The carrots, tangerines, and beets in this recipe are all rich in carotenoid compounds, such as lycopene. These nutrients neutralize free radicals and protect cells from oxidative stress. They selectively arrest cell growth and induce apoptosis in cancer cells without affecting normal, healthy cells.

SERVES ❷

½ cup carrot juice

½ cup tangerine juice

½ cup raw beet

½ cup green tea ice cubes

¼ cup hulled hemp seed

Combine all ingredients in a high-power blender or food processor and blend until smooth. Drink immediately.

Nutrition Facts *(per serving)*

Calories 170; Fat 9; Protein 8; Carbs 13; Fiber 2; Net Carbs 11

Research Study

C. Trejo-Solís, J. Pedraza-Chaverrí, M. Torres-Ramos, et al. (2013). Multiple molecular and cellular mechanisms of action of lycopene in cancer inhibition. *Evidence-Based Complementary and Alternative Medicine*, article ID 705121.

TANGERINE GREENS

*T*his fresh garden green smoothie has a sweet tangerine juice flavor and herbal green tea fragrance.

Lycopene is a carotenoid found in tomatoes, watermelon, guava, and grapefruit, which acts as an antioxidant, reducing free radicals and providing protection from developing cancer and reducing tumor growth.

SERVES **2**

½ cup tangerine juice

½ cup tomato

½ cup greens

½ cup green tea ice cubes

2 tablespoons chia seed

1 tablespoon lemon juice

Combine all ingredients in a high-power blender or food processor and blend until smooth. Drink immediately.

Nutrition Facts *(per serving)*

Calories 110; Fat 5; Protein 4; Carbs 14; Fiber 7; Net Carbs 7

Research Study

C. A. Thomson, N. R. Stendell-Hollis, C. L. Rock, et al. (2007). Plasma and dietary carotenoids are associated with reduced oxidative stress in women previously treated for breast cancer. *Cancer Epidemiology, Biomarkers and Prevention* 16 (10): 2008–15.

GRAPEFRUIT FROSTY

This frosty, golden smoothie has intense mandarin orange flavor that is mellowed by the sweet mango.

Nobiletin is a bioflavonoid found in citrus fruits, such as lemons, oranges, tangerines, and grapefruits. Nobiletin is an anti-inflammatory that suppresses metastasis of breast cancer.

SERVES ❷

1 mandarin orange

½ cup frozen mango

½ cup tangerine juice

½ cup green tea ice cubes

2 tablespoons hulled hemp seed

½ teaspoon rosemary leaf powder

Combine all ingredients in a high-power blender or food processor and blend until smooth. Drink immediately.

Nutrition Facts *(per serving)*

Calories 130; Fat 4; Protein 4; Carbs 20; Fiber 2; Net Carbs 18

Research Study

S. H. Baek, S. M. Kim, D. Nam, et al. (2012). Antimetastatic effect of nobiletin through the down-regulation of CXC chemokine receptor type 4 and matrix metallopeptidase-9. *Pharmaceutical Biology* 50 (10): 1210–18.

CARNOSOL DELIGHT

This smoothie is sweet and fruity with fresh herbal flavor and basil leaf fragrance.

Citrus fruits, such as the tangerine in this recipe, contain an antioxidant flavonoid called hesperidin that inhibits the growth and replication of breast cancer cells in laboratory studies.

SERVES ❷

½ cup tangerine juice

½ cup watermelon

½ cup green tea ice cubes

½ cup fresh basil leaves

2 tablespoons hulled hemp seed

¼ teaspoon rosemary leaf powder

Combine all ingredients in a high-power blender or food processor and blend until smooth. Drink immediately.

Nutrition Facts *(per serving)*

Calories 100; Fat 5; Protein 4; Carbs 10; Fiber 1; Net Carbs 9

Research Study

C. J. Lee, L. Wilson, M. A. Jordan, et al. (2009). Hesperidin suppressed proliferations of both human breast cancer and androgen-dependent prostate cancer cells. *Phytotherapy Research* 24 Suppl 1: S15–19.

PIPERINE PINEAPPLE

This is one of my favorite smoothies, as it has fresh and earthy basil and turmeric flavors in an exotic pineapple base.

Piperine is a bioactive component of black pepper that strongly inhibits proliferation of cancer cells and triggers the destruction of cancer cells.

SERVES ❷

½ cup tangerine juice

½ cup frozen pineapple

½ cup fresh basil leaves

½ cup green tea ice cubes

¼ cup hulled hemp seed

½ teaspoon turmeric powder

Pinch of fresh ground black pepper

Combine all ingredients in a high-power blender or food processor and blend until smooth. Drink immediately.

Nutrition Facts *(per serving)*

Calories 110; Fat 5; Protein 4; Carbs 14; Fiber 2; Net Carbs 12

Research Study

C. D. Doucette, A. L. Hilchie, R. Liwski, et al. (2012). Piperine, a dietary phytochemical, inhibits angiogenesis. *Journal of Nutritional Biochemistry* 24 (1): 231–39.

APPENDIX I: ALPHABETICAL LIST OF SMOOTHIES

Apple Smoothies

Apple Raspberry Tea 40

Blue Protein Power 45

Garden Greens 42

Golden Banana and Greens 44

Kale Apple Smash 43

Lemon Rosemary Tea 46

Quercetin Quencher 41

Apricot Smoothies

Apricot Green Tea 48

Cherry Apricot Frosty 57

Citrus Berry Punch 58

Golden Apricot Plum 56

Herbal Apricot 55

Lycopene Luster 59

Tart Apricot 49

Tart Apricot Grapefruit 60

Wild Blueberry Apricot 50

Blueberry Smoothies

Basil Berry Blend 67

Berry Burst Frosty 72

Blueberry Cherry 62

Blueberry Orange 70

Blue Watermelon Pom 63

Carnosic Berry 75

Holy Basil Elixir 77

Hot Ginger and Blueberry 66

Raspberry Lime 64

Strawberry Hemp Shake 71

Wild Blueberry and Banana 68

APPENDIX II: SMOOTHIE INGREDIENTS

Many fruits, vegetables, nuts, seeds, and nutrient-rich powders can be used in smoothies. This is a comprehensive list of the foods suitable for smoothies that have proven anti-breast cancer nutrients. Use this reference section to remind yourself of the array of ingredients that can be added to your smoothies and how to prep them.

Apples: Whole apples can be blended in high-power blenders. Cored apples will blend easily, and unfiltered apple juice can be added to any smoothie to add a sweet liquid base. Fresh, whole apples last for many weeks in a cool place, such as the refrigerator. Fresh apples can be used in smoothies; just remove the core and stem. Apples that have been chopped can be stored in a covered glass container for up to a week in the refrigerator.

Organic, unfiltered apple juice contains the antioxidant nutrients, such as quercetin, that are found in whole apples. Look for unsweetened apple juice and apple sauce in glass jars rather than plastic containers, some which may contain toxic phthalates.

Quercetin and triterpenoids help reduce inflammation and the growth of breast cancer cells. Unfiltered apple juice contains more of the nutrients from the skin, such as the triterpenoids, than clear, filtered juice.

Apricots—*See Stone Fruit*

Bananas: Bananas provide creamy texture and when frozen first, they give a smoothie a frosty, milkshake-like consistency. Bananas can be peeled and then the fruit can be frozen in waxed paper bags or BPA-free food storage bags.

Basil: Fresh basil leaves are available in the produce department of most grocery stores, and dried basil leaves are sold in bulk and in spice jars. Either can be used in smoothies. Fresh is preferable as it has fragrant, healthful oils that provide more concentrated nutrients, flavor, and fragrance than dried basil leaves.

Beets: Beets are rich in carotenoids, are widely available, and can be added to smoothies raw or cooked. Raw beets blend easily in high-power blenders and are preferable to canned beets, as cans are often lined with toxic plastics.

Berries: When picking fresh berries, be sure to rinse them well. Let them dry before freezing to avoid clumping and then store them in the freezer in a waxed-paper or BPA-free food storage bag. Buy organic juices and concentrates when possible.

- **Blackberries:** Fresh or frozen blackberries can be added to smoothies for their flavor and nutrients.

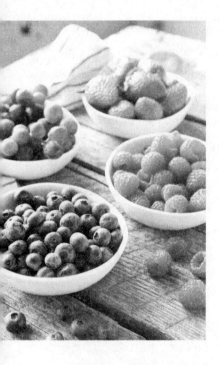

- **Blueberries:** Blueberries are sold in bags in the freezer section of most grocery stores specifically for smoothies. Whole, fresh, or frozen blueberries, blueberry juice, and blueberry nectar can be added directly to smoothies to add rich flavor and dense nutrients. Cultivated blueberries and wild blueberries contain phenolic antioxidants that have been found to act on breast cancer cells in several ways. Laboratory studies have proven their efficacy in reducing the growth, breakdown, and clearance of existing breast cancer cells.

- **Cranberries:** Fresh cranberries, cranberry juice, and cranberry juice concentrate add intense flavor and color to smoothies. The juice contains ellagic acid, a nutrient that has the ability to trigger apoptosis of breast cancer cells.

- **Grapes:** Most of the grape's nutrients are in the fruit's skin, so whole seedless grapes are an ideal smoothie ingredient. Dark-colored grape juice, especially unfiltered juice, contains the nutrient-rich skin pulp. Buy organic when possible. Seedless grapes can be used fresh or stored in an airtight container in the freezer. Frozen grapes create a frosty and rich texture in smoothies.

- **Raspberries:** Red raspberries specifically for use in smoothies are available in bags in the freezer section of the store.

- **Strawberries:** Fresh or frozen strawberries add sweet and fresh flavor to smoothies. Strawberries are one of the most highly sprayed crops, so it's essential to buy organic strawberries or grow your own. They should be rinsed and can be added whole to smoothies.

Wild Blueberries: Wild blueberries have a stronger flavor and color than cultivated blueberries. Wild blueberries are one of my favorite smoothie ingredients, as they contain concentrated amounts of the cancer-fighting antioxidants found in cultivated berries. They also have a richer flavor and brighter color. I buy them frozen and try to eat at least one-half cup per day of these nutrient powerhouses.

Blackberries—*See Berries*

Black Pepper—*See Spices*

Blueberries—*See Berries*

Cantaloupe—*See Melon*

Cardamom—*See Spices*

Carrots: Whole fresh carrots can be blended in high-power blenders and fresh carrot juice can be added to smoothies. Carrot juice can be made at home with a juicer or purchased in the refrigerator section of the grocery store. Carrot flavor blends well with citrus, as well as with greens and apples. Raw or cooked carrots, fresh homemade carrot juice, or store-bought carrot juice can be added to smoothies for sweet flavor and nutrients. Whole carrots and carrot juices are loaded with breast cancer-fighting carotenoids. Whole raw carrots can be blended in high powder blenders, or opt for carrot juice if you like a smoother texture without so much fiber in your smoothies.

Chia Seeds—*See Nuts and Seeds*

Cherries: Cherry juice and cherry concentrate are rich in nutrients and provide concentrated flavor in small quantities. Just a quarter cup of cherry juice provides sweet cherry flavor and fragrance to an entire smoothie. Frozen cherries come pre-pitted and are generally frozen at the peak of ripeness, so they're very sweet and easier to digest than unripe cherries. Choose your favorite variety, whether dark, sour, sweet, or tart, as they all provide an array of nutrients that support breast cancer recovery. Buy organic when possible. If you're using fresh cherries, be sure to remove the pit. Once the pit has been removed, you can freeze them for future use.

Cilantro—*See Greens*

Cinnamon: Ground cinnamon adds flavor and a little heat to smoothies. Ground or powdered cinnamon is available in the bulk department of the grocery store. Replace your cinnamon at least once a year, as the oils oxidize from light and oxygen, and it loses its health properties as well as its flavor over time.

Citrus: Citrus fruits contain an array of nutrients that are protective against breast cancer. They provide alpha carotene, beta-cryptoxanthin,

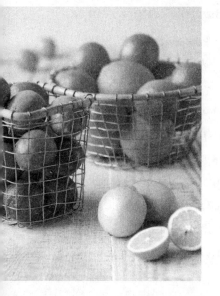

lycopene, lutein, and zeaxanthin, as well as the bioflavonoid nobiletin. Fresh citrus fruits, including oranges, grapefruit, tangerines, lemons, and limes, add sweet and tart flavor to smoothies. **One caveat with citrus and grapefruit is for those who are on aromatase inhibitors due to the cyp3A4 potential interaction. If you are on an aromatase inhibitor, avoid citrus.** Citrus peel is edible and can be blended; however, the skin may be too tough for most blenders and add an intense bitter flavor. You can either use your hands to peel the skin or use a knife to cut away the colorful, tough outer skin. The advantage of cutting away the peel is that you can leave much of the white pithy part of the peel intact. The pith is the part of the fruit that contains much of the bioflavonoids. Unpeeled fruit can be kept fresh in a cool, dry place for up to a week. Peeled fruit can be stored in waxed paper bags or BPA-free food storage bags in the refrigerator for about three days or in the freezer for months.

Edible essential citrus oils can be used in place of fresh citrus juice for their flavor, fragrance, and flavonoid content. Citrus fruits contain numerous compounds found to be therapeutically effective in supporting breast cancer recovery. Hesperidin, naringin, limonene, and nobiletin each provide specific anticancer actions against breast cancer. Citrus fruits also contain immune-boosting nutrients, such as vitamin C and bioflavonoids. Hesperetin, a flavanone glycoside found in citrus fruits, is cytotoxic to human breast carcinoma, which means that it causes apoptosis and is especially effective in reducing triple-negative breast cancer cells.

- **Grapefruit:** Grapefruit should be peeled first, then sections can be added to smoothies. The inner layer of the peel is rich in bioflavonoids, such as nobiletin. If you want to add peel for its health benefits, add two tablespoons of peel to your smoothie.
- **Lemon:** Peel the tough outer layer with a knife, leaving the white pithy inner part attached to the fruit, which is rich in bioflavonoids. Lemon juice can be made at home by cutting a lemon in half and poking the tines of a fork into the juicy part of the fruit and then twisting it to squeeze out the juice. Premade lemon juice is available at the grocery store. Santa Cruz and Lakewood brands sell organic citrus juice in glass bottles. Edible essential oils of lemons can be used in smoothies to add fragrance, flavor, and nutrients.

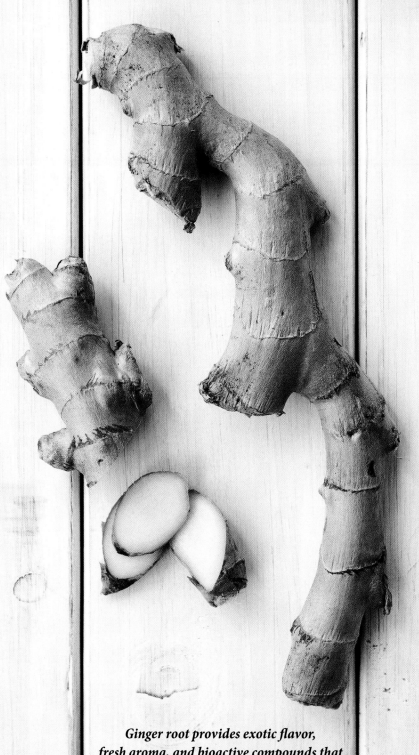

Ginger root provides exotic flavor, fresh aroma, and bioactive compounds that suppress breast cancer growth.

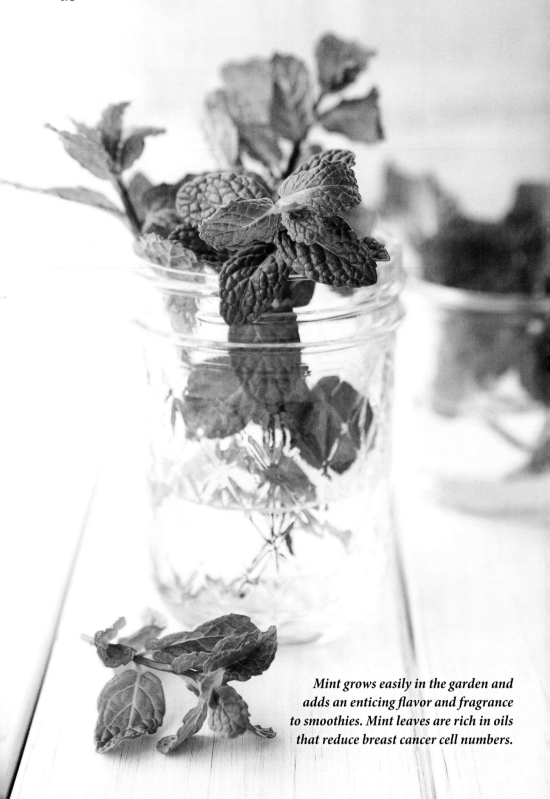

Mint grows easily in the garden and adds an enticing flavor and fragrance to smoothies. Mint leaves are rich in oils that reduce breast cancer cell numbers.

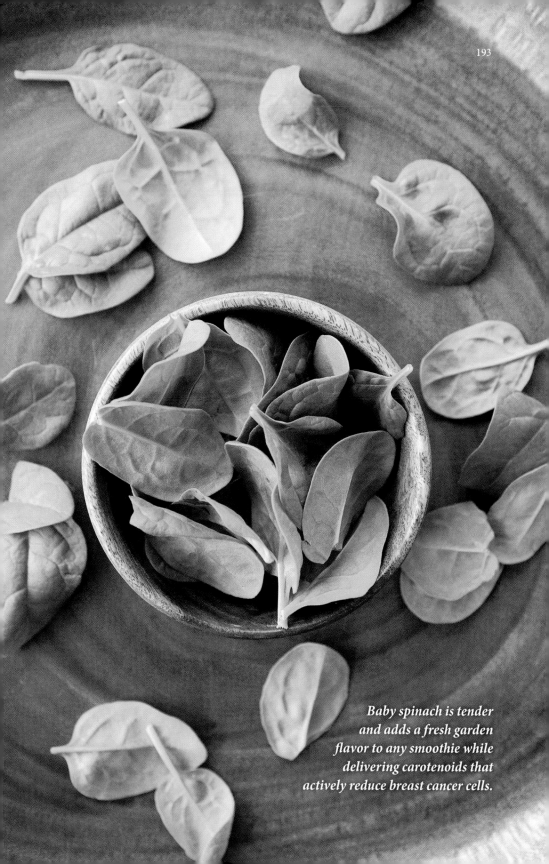

Baby spinach is tender and adds a fresh garden flavor to any smoothie while delivering carotenoids that actively reduce breast cancer cells.

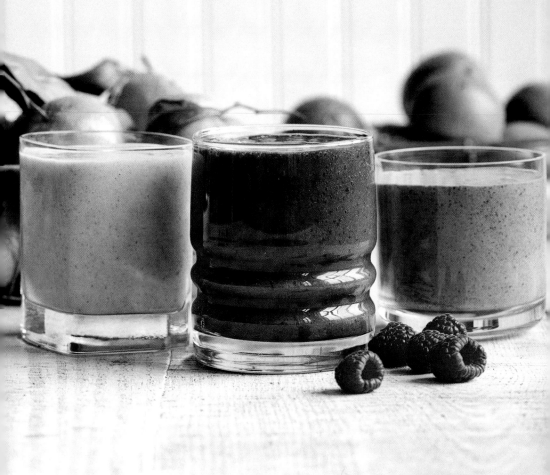

*Incorporate both fruits and vegetables in your smoothies as they each
provide concentrations of various anticancer nutrients.*

- **Lime:** Lime juice can be made at home by cutting a lime in half and poking the tines of a fork into the juicy part of the fruit and then twisting it to squeeze out the juice. Premade, organic, 100% lime juice in glass bottles is available in the grocery store. Santa Cruz and Lakewood brands sell organic citrus juice in glass. Fresh lime juice stays fresh in the refrigerator for weeks.

- **Orange:** Premade orange juice is available at the grocery store. Santa Cruz and Lakewood brands sell organic citrus juice in glass. Fresh orange juice stays fresh in the refrigerator for about a week. Oranges and orange juice give smoothies a fresh fruity base and blend with other fruits and vegetables, such as greens. Remember the caveat: Citrus is to be avoided by those who are on aromatase inhibitors due to the cyp3A4 potential interaction. If you are on an aromatase inhibitor, avoid citrus.

- **Tangerine:** Peeled tangerine segments can be added to smoothies. Tangerine skin contains concentrated phytochemicals that fight breast cancer. If you have a high-power blender, you can add a whole organic tangerine to your smoothie. Tangerine juice can be made at home, and fresh premade and bottled tangerine juice is available at the grocery store. Look for organic tangerine juice in glass bottles. Tangerine juice is sweet and a bit less acidic than orange juice.

Cloves—*See Spices*

Cocoa: Unsweetened cocoa powder provides antioxidants, cancer-reducing phytochemicals, and imparts rich chocolate flavor without sugar.

Coconut

- **Coconut milk:** Coconut milk is a creamy, low-sugar, vegan, liquid smoothie base that provides protein and fiber. It's available in cartons that do not require refrigeration until opened, called aspect boxes. Buy organic, non-GMO products when possible.

- **Coconut water:** Coconut water is the clear liquid from inside young coconuts that has a light coconut flavor. It is rich in sodium, magnesium, calcium, phosphorus, and especially potassium, each of which supports hydration. The light coconut flavor pairs well with most fruit combinations. Coconut water is available in most grocery stores. Look for coconut waters that are organic, non-GMO, and bottled fresh, rather than being made from concentrate.

- **Cultured coconut milk:** Cultured coconut milk products contain "culture," which are probiotic organisms. They provide the much-needed microbes that metabolize food nutrients, such as breast cancer-fighting antioxidants.

Cranberries—*See Berries*

Dairy Alternatives: Dairy foods should be avoided because of their natural and possibly synthetic (bovine growth injections) hormone content. Dairy alternatives that can be used in smoothies include nut milks (almond, cashew, hazelnut), rice milk, hemp milk, and coconut milk.

Garlic: Garlic has a strong flavor and a sulfurous smell, so start with one clove, blend, and taste. If you want more garlic flavor, add another clove and work your way up to the right level of heat and garlic bite. Peel the papery skin from each clove before adding them to smoothies. Fresh garlic is available year-round in the produce department of the grocery store. Dried garlic granules and dried garlic powder are also available in the spice and bulk sections of the grocery store, but fresh is preferable, as the oils in the cloves lose some of their medicinal properties when dried.

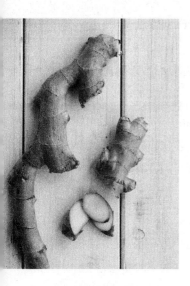

Ginger: Whole, fresh ginger root is found in the produce section of the grocery store. Ginger root juice adds an Asian flair and a little heat to smoothies. Ginger root juice, pickled slices, and ground ginger can be used in smoothies. High-power blenders can pulverize the woody tuber of fresh ginger. However, if your blender has a hard time with tough fibers such as this, you can extract the juice by squeezing chopped fresh ginger root through a garlic press. The papery outer skin is edible.

Grapefruit—*See Citrus*

Grapes—*See Berries*

Greens: Dark leafy greens, such as kale, baby spinach, cilantro, chard, and Italian parsley, can be blended into smoothies. Buy organic when possible, as organic greens contain higher levels of fat-soluble vitamins. Use the stems and the leaves and give them a thorough rinse. Wash the unused leaves and wrap them, while still wet, in a clean cloth towel and store in the crisper drawer of your refrigerator for up to a week.

- **Cilantro:** Cilantro leaves have an intense flavor that most people either love or hate. I happen to love it. But these tiny, oil-rich leaves change the flavor of a smoothie quickly, so add just a tablespoon at a time and taste before adding more so you can adjust the flavor to your palate. Wash the leaves and wrap them, while still wet, in a clean cloth towel and store in the crisper drawer of your refrigerator for up to a week.
- **Kale:** Fresh kale leaves and other greens are delicious blended with apples, lemons, and other citrus fruits. Buy organic kale when possible,

as organic greens contain higher levels of fat-soluble vitamins. Fresh greens have a short shelf life. Wash the leaves and wrap them, while still wet, in a clean cloth towel and store in the crisper drawer of your refrigerator for up to a week.

- **Spinach:** Fresh and even frozen spinach is rich in carotenoids and blends well with stone fruit, apples, citrus flavors, and carrots. Baby spinach is especially tender and blends easily, making it an ideal smoothie ingredient.

Green Tea: Brew loose leaf or bagged green tea following the package instructions. Steep for just under two minutes and let cool before adding to smoothies. By removing the tea leaves from the brewed tea at this point, you retain the maximum amount of the cancer-protecting catechins without extracting the undesirable compounds, such as bitter tannins and excess caffeine. Decaf green tea can also be used, as it provides all of the same nutrients as caffeinated green tea.

Brewed tea can be poured into ice trays to make tea cubes. Ice cube trays made from 100% silicone, such as the Lekue brand, are nontoxic and easy to bend, allowing the cubes to be removed easily from the tray. The cubes can be popped out of their trays and into waxed paper bags or BPA-free food storage bags and placed in the freezer for quick use in smoothies. I prefer freezing tea, rather than brewing tea each time I want to add some to a smoothie. The cubes will last indefinitely in the freezer and they add a frosty texture to smoothies.

Green tea, when brewed properly, provides powerful catechins with preventive and therapeutic properties.

Epigallocatechin-gallate (EGCG) is a catechin in green tea that may inhibit breast cancer progression by blocking angiogenesis. Recently, Romanian researchers have shown that EGCG suppresses the growth, migration, and invasion of human breast cancer cells. The research shows that catechins from green tea reduce the growth and spread of breast cancer cells; however, the amount of tea needed to produce these effects is still being studied. Until studies provide more specific recommendations, aim for one to two cups of green tea per day.

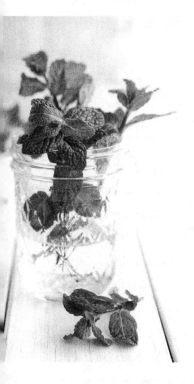

Holy Basil: Tulsi, which is also known as holy basil, is a dietary herb used for its multiple beneficial pharmacologic properties, including anti-cancer activity. Dried holy basil is available from the bulk spice section of many grocery stores. The dried leaves can be added directly to smoothies or, if your blender has a hard time breaking down dried herbs, they can be ground first in a coffee grinder. Ground holy basil can be stored in an airtight container in the freezer for months. Holy basil plants are often available at garden stores and can be grown in your garden or in a pot on a porch. Fresh holy basil leaves are available in the produce department of many specialty markets, farmer's markets, and ethnic markets.

Hulled Hemp Seed—*See Nuts and Seeds*

Lemon—*See Citrus*

Lime—*See Citrus*

Mango—*See Stone Fruit*

Melon

- **Cantaloupe:** Melons, such as cantaloupe, can be added fresh or frozen. Just remove the rind and add the melon flesh with the seeds. Fresh melon can be stored for months in an airtight container in the freezer. High-power blenders can power through frozen melon chunks, and they give smoothies a frosty texture.

- **Watermelon:** Frozen watermelon provides a lush, frosty texture. Watermelon is rich in carotenoids and adds a sweet, distinctive flavor that pairs well with berries and other melon. To prepare watermelon for smoothies, remove the rind and cut the melon into large chunks. Choose seedless watermelon if you prefer an even texture without seed bits in your smoothies. Once the rind is removed, watermelon chunks can be frozen to keep them fresh.

Nectar: Fruit nectars are similar to juice but contain more pulp and have a richer flavor and more fiber. Many fruit nectars are available in grocery stores, such as blueberry, apricot, peach, and mango.

Nuts and Seeds

- **Chia seeds:** Chia are tiny seeds that can be purchased at the grocery store and online. When blended with liquid, they act as an emulsifier by thickening and keeping ingredients from separating. Chia seed can be added directly to smoothies or ground in a coffee grinder into a powder. Whole and ground chia seeds can be stored in an airtight container in the freezer for months. Frozen chia, whether in whole seed or ground powder form, will stay fresh longer than at room temperature. Chia seeds are a rich source of nutrition and contain 2.5 grams of protein and 5 grams of fiber per tablespoon. They also contain inflammation-reducing omega fatty acids, providing 2,400 milligrams (mg) of omega-3 fatty acids and 800 mg of omega-6 fatty acids in each tablespoon.

- **Hulled hemp seed:** Hulled hemp seed and hemp protein powder can be purchased in most stores and online. Bob's Red Mill line of products offers both, and they are always fresh and widely available. Hemp products are vegan and rich in protein and omega fatty acids. Hulled hemp seed blends so well in smoothies that it creates a cream-like texture.
- **Sunflower seeds:** Sunflower seeds blend easily and create a rich texture and nutty flavor in smoothies. Nuts and seeds can be stored in the refrigerator in an airtight container to reduce exposure to light and oxygen, which cause rancidity. They stay fresh for months when frozen.

Oats: Rolled oats can be added to smoothies and provide breast cancer protective dietary lignans. Bob's Red Mill brand offers both organic and gluten-free rolled oats in large bags, which can be purchased online, in most grocery stores, and at Costco.

Oranges—*See Citrus*

Papaya: It's possible to use the entire papaya in a smoothie if it is organic. Chunks of peeled and seeded flesh can be frozen, as frozen fruit blends well and gives smoothies a rich, frosty texture. Lime pairs exceptionally well with this tropical fruit.

Peaches—*See Stone Fruit*

Pineapple: Fresh pineapple can be purchased in the produce department of most grocery stores. When purchasing a pineapple, choose one that is as ripe as possible. Ripe pineapple has a strong pineapple scent and the leaves sprouting out of the top release easily when plucked. To prep fresh pineapple, remove the skin with a knife, as well as the top and the bottom, then slice the whole fruit. The fresh fruit can then be added to smoothies or frozen for future use. Canned pineapple is available but not recommended, as the cans are lined with plastics that release phthalates into acidic foods such as pineapple.

Plum—*See Stone Fruit*

Pomegranate: Whole pomegranates are available seasonally in the produce section of the grocery store. They can be expensive, and the seeds (arils) that contain the juice need to be removed from the fruit to be used in smoothies. Pomegranate arils are available in the freezer section of the grocery store. Organic 100% pomegranate juice and pomegranate juice concentrate are available in glass jars. The juice stays fresh for about a week once opened and can be frozen into cubes to keep fresh.

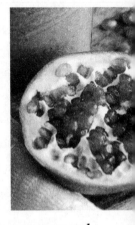

Pomegranate fruit seeds, which are called arils, and their juice are sweet and tannic additions to smoothies. They contain powerful nutrients that inhibit breast cancer cells. Polyphenols found in the oils, skins, arils, concentrate, and juice of pomegranate exhibit growth-inhibiting effects on breast cancer cells. Pomegranate seeds contain phytochemicals that interfere with carcinogenesis, meaning that they reduce not only inflammation but also the growth and spread of breast cancer cells. Pomegranate enhances chemotherapy and directly reduces metastasis and angiogenesis.

Probiotic Powders: Probiotics are sold in several forms, including capsules, powders, and liquids. Powdered products have a longer shelf life than liquid products and mix well into smoothies. Look for probiotic products that contain *Lactobacillus acidophilus.*

Protein Powders: Organic, vegan protein powders are an excellent source of powdered protein. They also help to thicken and emulsify smoothies. Look for pea or rice protein powders. Protein powders are sold as plain or flavored, such as vanilla. Read the label to make sure you aren't getting too much sugar when you opt for a flavored protein powder.

Prunes—*See Stone Fruit*

Raspberries—*See Berries*

Rosemary: Fresh, dried, and ground rosemary can all be used in smoothies. Dried whole rosemary leafs look like pine needles. Ground rosemary leaves may be coarsely or finely ground. The finely ground powder works best in smoothies, as it softens and blends easily. Fresh rosemary contains concentrated amounts of phenolic compounds that reduce inflammation and inhibit breast cancer cell growth.

Spices

- **Black pepper:** Fresh ground pepper is a powerhouse of breast cancer-fighting nutrients and potassium. Buy dried black peppercorns, which can be found in bulk and in jars in the spice section of the grocery store. Use a pepper mill to grind the peppercorns as needed. The nutrient-rich oils are well preserved in the peppercorns and are released once they're ground.
- **Cardamom:** Cardamom pods and ground cardamom powder can be purchased from the bulk section of the grocery store. They provide a

heady aroma and flavor to smoothies and can be stored for up to a year
in an airtight glass container.

- **Cloves:** Whole cloves and ground cloves are sold in spice jars and in
  bulk. Ground clove powder blends well in smoothies. Use only small
  amounts as the oils impart a strong flavor and fragrance. Whole cloves
  can be stored in a glass jar for up to a year. Ground cloves stay fresh for
  about six months in an airtight container.
- **Turmeric:** Fresh turmeric root is found in the produce section of the
  grocery store. Dried turmeric powder and ground turmeric root are
  available in jars and in the bulk spice section of the grocery store. The
  golden yellow powder can stain countertops and clothing, so handle
  it carefully. When stored in an airtight container, it will stay fresh for
  months.
- **Vanilla:** Vanilla extract adds a lot of flavor without adding many
  calories or any sugar to smoothies. Whole vanilla beans can be used
  in high-power blenders.

Stone Fruit: Stone fruit are generally sweet and add intense flavor. They
contain valuable breast cancer-fighting nutrients to smoothies. Apricots, mangoes, and peaches contain antioxidant carotenoids that can reduce precancerous cell changes that may lead to the formation of breast tumors. Whole, fresh
(pitted) stone fruit and their juice and nectar can be used in smoothies. Their
flavors combine well with other fruits, berries, and even greens.

- **Apricots:** Fresh apricots are available in the produce department of
  most grocery stores during the summer months in the United States.
  The pit must be removed, but the skin can be blended. Apricot nectar
  is similar to juice but contains more apricot pulp and has a richer
  flavor and more fiber. Look for nectars and juices that are in glass
  bottles, such as the Knudsen brand.

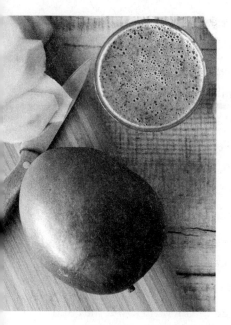

- **Mango:** Look for mangoes that have orange to red skin color, which indicates ripeness. Young mangoes are green and turn yellow as they ripen, then patches of red develop and they dent like an avocado when pressed. Fresh mangoes can be added to smoothies once the pit is removed. If you use a high-power blender, use the skin too, because it contains concentrated bioactives that inhibit breast cancer cell growth. Frozen mango that has been peeled, pitted, chopped, and frozen is available in the freezer section of grocery stores. The fruit is frozen when it is at its ripest and sweet, and there is no mess to clean up as there is when prepping fresh mango at home. Also, fresh mangoes are not always ripe in grocery stores. Mango gives smoothies a creamy and frosty texture with rich tropical flavor. Since mangoes are being genetically modified and carry a higher residue of agricultural chemicals in their skin and flesh, it's important to buy organic. They are rich in fiber, carotenoids, and natural plant compounds that cause apoptosis (cancer cell destruction) in breast cancer studies.

- **Peaches:** Peaches are a stone fruit and must have their pit removed before blending, but the skin can be left on, as it blends easily. Once pitted, the fruit can be used in a smoothie or frozen for later use. Stone fruit is often heavily sprayed with agricultural chemicals. To avoid chemical residue on stone fruit, look for peaches that are labeled as organic, which ensures that no chemical sprays have been used in the growing of the fruit. Whole fresh peaches provide rich, sweet flavor and pair well with berries and other fruits, as well as greens. Peach nectar is an ideal liquid smoothie base as it is rich in pulp, flavor, and anticancer nutrients. Frozen peach slices are available in the freezer section of the grocery store and are sold specifically for smoothies. They're sweet and delicious because they are frozen when they're at their peak ripeness. They are a rich source of carotenoids, anthocyanins, and vitamin C, which all play a role in breast cancer prevention and healing.

- **Plums:** Fresh plums must have their pit removed before blending. The skin will blend easily and the pitted fruit can be frozen.
- **Prunes:** Prunes are simply dried plums. The advantage of using dried plums rather than fresh is that they have a longer shelf life. They are pitted before drying so they're ready to add to smoothies, and they add sweetness, flavor, fiber, and active compounds that help reduce breast tumors.

Strawberries—*See Berries*

Sunflower Seeds—*See Nuts and Seeds*

Tangerine—*See Citrus*

Tart Cherries—*See Berries*

Tomato: Fresh organic tomatoes of all varieties provide carotenoids that reduce oxidative stress. Organic tomatoes have a higher concentration of these nutrients than nonorganic.

Turmeric—*See Spices*

Vanilla—*See Spices*

Water: Proper hydration is critical to the healing process. Aim for eight (8-ounce) glasses of pure water each day. Pure water can either be tap water that has been purified through a solid carbon filter or bottled filtered water in glass bottles (not plastic). Purified water can be used as the liquid base in smoothies and can also be used to make ice cubes, which can replace the green tea ice cubes in these recipes.

Watermelon—*See Melon*

Wild Blueberries—*See Berries*

APPENDIX III: GROCERY LISTS OF SMOOTHIE INGREDIENTS BY BREAST CANCER SUBTYPE

The following grocery lists are specific to common breast cancer subtypes. These are provided as a reminder of the foods discussed throughout the book and for inspiration as we tend to eat the same foods each day.

Consider scanning the lists that fit your diagnosis before grocery shopping, and adding a few new items to your cart each time you grocery shop. This way you can gradually introduce healing foods into your diet without having to make dramatic dietary changes.

The lists include the foods that provide support for all types of breast cancer, and additionally, the foods that are most effective for each of the specific subtypes.

For example, groups of foods like berries, stone fruit, and greens are supportive for all subtypes, but foods such as probiotics, hemp seed, and green tea were found to have a particular affinity for some subtypes. So there are crossovers and yet differences in each list.

Use the lists as references to remind you of the smoothie ingredients with the most benefit for your individual needs.

I hope that they inspire you to fill your kitchen with foods that help you heal.

Smoothie Ingredient Grocery List for BRCA 1 and BRCA 2 Subtypes

❏ Apples

❏ Apricots

❏ Bananas

❏ Basil

❏ Black cherries

❏ Black pepper

❏ Blackberries

❏ Black grapes

❏ Black raspberries

❏ Blueberries

❏ Cantaloupe

❏ Cardamom

❏ Carrots

❏ Carrot juice

❏ Cherries

❏ Chia

❏ Cilantro

❏ Cinnamon

❏ Cranberries

❏ Cranberry juice

❏ Garlic

❏ Ginger root

❏ Grapefruit

❏ Grapes

❏ Green leaf lettuce

❏ Holy basil

❏ Honeydew

❏ Kale

❏ Kumquats

❏ Lemons

❏ Limes

❏ Mango

❏ Nectarines

❏ Oranges

❏ Peach nectar

❏ Peaches

❏ Pears

❏ Pineapple

❏ Plums

❏ Pomegranate

❏ Powdered cloves

❏ Protein powder

❏ Prunes

❏ Raspberries

❏ Red leaf lettuce

❏ Romaine lettuce

❏ Rosemary

❏ Spinach

❏ Strawberries

❏ Swiss chard

❏ Tangerines

❏ Turmeric

❏ Unsweetened cocoa powder

❏ Vanilla

❏ Watermelon

❏ Wild blueberries

❏ White tea

Smoothie Ingredient Grocery List for
ER+ (Estrogen Receptor Positive) Subtype

❑ Apples

❑ Apricots

❑ Bananas

❑ Basil

❑ Beets

❑ Black cherries

❑ Black pepper

❑ Blackberries

❑ Blueberries

❑ Cabbage

❑ Cantaloupe

❑ Cardamom

❑ Carrots

❑ Carrot juice

❑ Cherries

❑ Chia

❑ Cilantro

❑ Cinnamon

❑ Cultured coconut milk

❑ Garlic

❑ Ginger root

❑ Grapefruit

❑ Grapes

❑ Green leaf lettuce

❑ Guava

❑ Holy basil

❑ Honeydew

❑ Kale

❑ Kumquats

❑ Lemons

❑ Limes

❑ Mango

❑ Nectarines

❑ Oranges

❑ Papaya

❑ Peaches

❑ Pineapple

❑ Plums

❑ Pomegranate

❑ Powdered cloves

❑ Probiotic powder

❑ Protein powder

❑ Prunes

❑ Raspberries

❑ Red leaf lettuce

❑ Romaine lettuce

❑ Rosemary

❑ Spinach

❑ Strawberries

❑ Swiss chard

❑ Tangerines

❑ Turmeric

❑ Unsweetened cocoa powder

❑ Vanilla

❑ Walnuts

❑ Watermelon

❑ Watercress

❑ White pepper

❑ White tea

❑ Wild strawberries

Smoothie Ingredient Grocery List for
ER- (Estrogen Receptor Negative) Subtype

❑ Apples

❑ Apricots

❑ Avocado

❑ Bananas

❑ Basil

❑ Beet greens

❑ Beets

❑ Black cherries

❑ Black pepper

❑ Blackberries

❑ Blueberries

❑ Butterhead lettuce

❑ Cantaloupe

❑ Cardamom

❑ Carrots

❑ Carrot juice

❑ Cherries

❑ Cilantro

❑ Cinnamon

❑ Chia

❑ Cranberries

❑ Cranberry juice

❑ Garlic

❑ Ginger root

❑ Grapes

❑ Grapefruit

❑ Green leaf lettuce

❑ Holy basil

❑ Honeydew

❑ Hulled hemp seed

❑ Kale

❑ Kumquats

❑ Lemons

❑ Limes

❑ Mango

❑ Nectarines

❑ Oranges

❑ Papaya

❑ Peach nectar

❑ Peaches

❑ Pineapple

❑ Plums

❑ Pomegranate

❑ Powdered cloves

❑ Protein powder

❑ Prunes

❑ Raspberries

❑ Red leaf lettuce

❑ Romaine lettuce

❑ Rosemary

❑ Spinach

❑ Strawberries

❑ Swiss chard

❑ Tangerines

❑ Turmeric

❑ Unsweetened cocoa powder

❑ Vanilla

❑ Watermelon

❑ White tea

Smoothie Ingredient Grocery List for HER2+ (Human Epidermal Growth Factor Receptor 2 Positive) Subtype

❏ Apples

❏ Apricots

❏ Avocado

❏ Bananas

❏ Basil

❏ Beet greens

❏ Beets

❏ Black cherries

❏ Black pepper

❏ Blackberries

❏ Blueberries

❏ Bok choy

❏ Cantaloupe

❏ Cardamom

❏ Carrots

❏ Carrot juice

❏ Cherries

❏ Chia

❏ Chinese cabbage

❏ Cilantro

❏ Cinnamon

❏ Collard greens

❏ Cranberries

❏ Cranberry juice

❏ Garlic

❏ Ginger root

❏ Grapefruit

❏ Grapes

❏ Green leaf lettuce

❏ Holy basil

❏ Honeydew

❏ Kale

❏ Kumquats

❏ Lemons

❏ Limes

❏ Mango

❏ Mustard greens

❏ Nectarines

❏ Oranges

❏ Papaya

❏ Peaches

❏ Pineapple

❏ Pomegranate

❏ Powdered cloves

❏ Plums

❏ Probiotic powder

❏ Protein powder

❏ Raspberries

❏ Red leaf lettuce

❏ Romaine lettuce

❏ Rosemary

❏ Spinach

❏ Strawberries

❏ Swiss chard

❏ Tangerines

❏ Turmeric

❏ Unsweetened cocoa powder

❏ Vanilla

❏ Watercress

❏ Watermelon

❏ White pepper

❏ White tea

Smoothie Ingredient Grocery List for HER2- (Human Epidermal Growth Factor Receptor 2 Negative) Subtype

- ❏ Apples
- ❏ Apricots
- ❏ Bananas
- ❏ Basil
- ❏ Beets
- ❏ Black cherries
- ❏ Black pepper
- ❏ Blackberries
- ❏ Blueberries
- ❏ Bok choy
- ❏ Cantaloupe
- ❏ Cardamom
- ❏ Carrots
- ❏ Carrot juice
- ❏ Cherries
- ❏ Chia
- ❏ Chinese cabbage
- ❏ Cilantro
- ❏ Cinnamon
- ❏ Cranberries
- ❏ Cranberry juice
- ❏ Cultured almond milk
- ❏ Garlic
- ❏ Ginger root
- ❏ Grapes
- ❏ Grapefruit
- ❏ Green leaf lettuce
- ❏ Holy basil
- ❏ Honeydew
- ❏ Kale
- ❏ Kumquats
- ❏ Lemons
- ❏ Limes
- ❏ Mango
- ❏ Mustard greens
- ❏ Nectarines
- ❏ Oranges
- ❏ Papaya
- ❏ Peaches
- ❏ Pineapple
- ❏ Plums
- ❏ Pomegranate
- ❏ Powdered cloves
- ❏ Protein powder
- ❏ Raspberries
- ❏ Red leaf lettuce
- ❏ Romaine lettuce
- ❏ Rosemary
- ❏ Spinach
- ❏ Strawberries
- ❏ Swiss chard
- ❏ Tangerines
- ❏ Turmeric
- ❏ Unsweetened cocoa powder
- ❏ Vanilla
- ❏ Watercress
- ❏ Watermelon
- ❏ White pepper
- ❏ White tea

Smoothie Ingredient Grocery List for Premenopausal Subtype

❏ Apples

❏ Apricots

❏ Bananas

❏ Basil

❏ Beets

❏ Bitter orange

❏ Black cherries

❏ Black pepper

❏ Blackberries

❏ Blueberries

❏ Cabbage

❏ Cantaloupe

❏ Cardamom

❏ Carrots

❏ Cherries

❏ Chia

❏ Cilantro

❏ Cinnamon

❏ Cranberries

❏ Cranberry juice

❏ Cultured coconut milk

❏ Garlic

❏ Ginger root

❏ Grapes

❏ Grapefruit

❏ Green leaf lettuce

❏ Holy Basil

❏ Honeydew

❏ Kale

❏ Kumquats

❏ Lemons

❏ Limes

❏ Mandarin orange

❏ Mango

❏ Nectarines

❏ Oranges

❏ Papaya

❏ Peaches

❏ Pineapple

❏ Plums

❏ Pomegranate

❏ Powdered cloves

❏ Probiotic powder

❏ Protein powder

❏ Prunes

❏ Raspberries

❏ Red leaf lettuce

❏ Romaine lettuce

❏ Rosemary

❏ Spinach

❏ Strawberries

❏ Swiss chard

❏ Tangerines

❏ Turmeric

❏ Unsweetened coconut water

❏ Vanilla

❏ Watermelon

❏ Watercress

❏ White tea

Smoothie Ingredient Grocery List for Postmenopausal Subtype

❑ Almond butter

❑ Apples

❑ Apricots

❑ Avocado

❑ Bananas

❑ Basil

❑ Beets

❑ Black cherries

❑ Black pepper

❑ Blackberries

❑ Blueberries

❑ Cantaloupe

❑ Cardamom

❑ Carrots

❑ Carrot juice

❑ Cherries

❑ Chia seeds

❑ Cilantro

❑ Cinnamon

❑ Cranberries

❑ Cranberry juice

❑ Garlic

❑ Ginger root

❑ Grapes

❑ Grapefruit

❑ Green leaf lettuce

❑ Guava

❑ Holy basil

❑ Honeydew

❑ Hulled hemp seed

❑ Kale

❑ Kumquats

❑ Lemons

❑ Limes

❑ Mango

❑ Mango nectar

❑ Nectarines

❑ Orange juice

❑ Oranges

❑ Papaya

❑ Peach nectar

❑ Peaches

❑ Pineapple

❑ Plums

❑ Pomegranate

❑ Powdered cloves

❑ Protein powder

❑ Prunes

❑ Raspberries

❑ Red leaf lettuce

❑ Romaine lettuce

❑ Rosemary

❑ Spinach

❑ Strawberries

❑ Sunflower seeds

❑ Swiss chard

❑ Tangerines

❑ Tomato

❑ Turmeric

❑ Unsweetened cocoa powder

❑ Watermelon

❑ White Tea

Smoothie Ingredient Grocery List for PR+ (Progesterone Receptor Positive) Subtype

❏ Almond milk

❏ Apples

❏ Apricots

❏ Avocado

❏ Bananas

❏ Basil

❏ Beets

❏ Black cherries

❏ Black pepper

❏ Blackberries

❏ Blueberries

❏ Cantaloupe

❏ Cardamom

❏ Carrots

❏ Carrot juice

❏ Cherries

❏ Chia

❏ Cilantro

❏ Cinnamon

❏ Cranberries

❏ Cranberry juice

❏ Cultured almond milk

❏ Cultured coconut milk

❏ Garlic

❏ Grapefruit

❏ Grapes

❏ Green leaf lettuce

❏ Hemp milk

❏ Holy basil

❏ Honeydew

❏ Hulled hemp seed

❏ Kale

❏ Kumquats

❏ Lemons

❏ Limes

❏ Mango

❏ Nectarines

❏ Oranges

❏ Papaya

❏ Peach nectar

❏ Peaches

❏ Pineapple

❏ Plums

❏ Pomegranate

❏ Pomelo

❏ Powdered cloves

❏ Protein powder

❏ Prunes

❏ Raspberries

❏ Red leaf lettuce

❏ Romaine lettuce

❏ Rosemary

❏ Spinach

❏ Strawberries

❏ Swiss chard

❏ Tangerines

❏ Turmeric

❏ Unsweetened cocoa powder

❏ Vanilla

❏ Watermelon

❏ White tea

Smoothie Ingredient Grocery List for
PR- (Progesterone Receptor Negative) Subtype

❏ Almonds

❏ Apples

❏ Apricots

❏ Avocado

❏ Bananas

❏ Basil

❏ Beets

❏ Black cherries

❏ Black pepper

❏ Blackberries

❏ Blueberries

❏ Cantaloupe

❏ Cardamom

❏ Carrots

❏ Carrot juice

❏ Cherries

❏ Chia

❏ Cilantro

❏ Cinnamon

❏ Cranberries

❏ Cranberry juice

❏ Garlic

❏ Ginger root

❏ Grapes

❏ Grapefruit

❏ Green leaf lettuce

❏ Holy basil

❏ Honeydew

❏ Hulled hemp seed

❏ Kale

❏ Kumquats

❏ Lemons

❏ Limes

❏ Mango

❏ Nectarines

❏ Oranges

❏ Papaya

❏ Peach nectar

❏ Peaches

❏ Pineapple

❏ Plums

❏ Pomegranate

❏ Powdered cloves

❏ Protein powder

❏ Prunes

❏ Raspberries

❏ Red leaf lettuce

❏ Romaine lettuce

❏ Rosemary

❏ Sesame seeds

❏ Spinach

❏ Strawberries

❏ Swiss chard

❏ Tangerines

❏ Turmeric

❏ Unsweetened cocoa
   powder

❏ Vanilla

❏ Watermelon

❏ White tea

Smoothie Ingredient Grocery List for TNBC (Triple-Negative Breast Cancer) Subtype

- ❑ Apple
- ❑ Apricots
- ❑ Bananas
- ❑ Basil
- ❑ Beets
- ❑ Black cherries
- ❑ Black cherry juice
- ❑ Black pepper
- ❑ Blackberries
- ❑ Black cherry juice
- ❑ Blueberries
- ❑ Cantaloupe
- ❑ Cardamom
- ❑ Carrots
- ❑ Carrot juice
- ❑ Cherries
- ❑ Chia
- ❑ Cilantro
- ❑ Cinnamon
- ❑ Cranberries
- ❑ Cranberry juice
- ❑ Garlic
- ❑ Ginger root
- ❑ Grapefruit
- ❑ Grapes
- ❑ Green leaf lettuce
- ❑ Green tea
- ❑ Holy basil
- ❑ Honeydew
- ❑ Hulled hemp seed
- ❑ Kale
- ❑ Kumquats
- ❑ Lemons
- ❑ Limes
- ❑ Mango
- ❑ Nectarines
- ❑ Oranges
- ❑ Papaya
- ❑ Peach nectar
- ❑ Peaches
- ❑ Pineapple
- ❑ Plums
- ❑ Pomegranate
- ❑ Pomelo
- ❑ Powdered cloves
- ❑ Protein powder
- ❑ Prunes
- ❑ Raspberries
- ❑ Red leaf lettuce
- ❑ Romaine lettuce
- ❑ Rosemary
- ❑ Spinach
- ❑ Strawberries
- ❑ Swiss chard
- ❑ Tangerines
- ❑ Tomatoes
- ❑ Turmeric
- ❑ Unsweetened cocoa powder
- ❑ Vanilla
- ❑ Watermelon
- ❑ White tea
- ❑ Wild blueberries

REFERENCES

ALUMINUM

Darbre, P. D., D. Pugazhendhi, and F. Mannello. (2011). Aluminum and human breast diseases. *Journal of Inorganic Biochemistry* 105 (11): 1484–88.

Mannello, F., D. Ligi, and M. Canale. (2013). Aluminum, carbonyls and cytokines in human nipple aspirate fluids: Possible relationship between inflammation, oxidative stress and breast cancer microenvironment. *Journal of Inorganic Biochemistry* 128:250–56.

Romanowicz-Makowska, H., E. Forma, M. Bryś, et al. (2011). Concentration of cadmium, nickel and aluminum in female breast cancer. *Polish Journal of Pathology* 62 (4): 257–61.

APPLES

Bulzomi, P., P. Galluzzo, A. Bolli, et al. (2012). The pro-apoptotic effect of quercetin in cancer cell lines requires ERβ-dependent signals. *Journal of Cellular Physiology* 227 (5): 1891–98.

Delphi, L., H. Sepehri, M. R. Khorramizadeh, et al. (2015). Pectic-oligosaccharides from apples induce apoptosis and cell cycle arrest in MDA-MB-231 cells, a model of human breast cancer. *Asian Pacific Organization for Cancer Prevention* 16 (13): 5265–71.

He, X., Y. Wang, H. Hu, et al. (2012). In vitro and in vivo antimammary tumor activities and mechanisms of the apple total triterpenoids. *Journal of Agricultural and Food Chemistry* 60 (37): 9430–36.

Huang, C., S. Y. Lee, C. L. Lin, et al. (2013). Co-treatment with quercetin and 1,2,3,4,6-penta-O-galloyl-β-D-glucose causes cell cycle arrest and apoptosis in human breast cancer MDA-MB-231 and AU565 cells. *Journal of Agricultural and Food Chemistry* 61 (26): 6430–45.

Reagan-Shaw, S., D. Eggert, H. Mukhtar, et al. (2010). Antiproliferative effects of apple peel extract against cancer cells. *Nutrition and Cancer* 62 (4): 517–24.

Sangai, N. P., R. J. Verma, and M. H. Trivedi. (2012). Testing the efficacy of quercetin in mitigating bisphenol A toxicity in liver and kidney of mice. *Toxicology and Industrial Health* 30 (7): 581–97.

APRICOT

Bhuvaneswari, V., and S. Nagini. (2005). Lycopene: A review of its potential as an anticancer agent. *Current Medicinal Chemistry Anticancer Agents* 5 (6): 627–35.

Kabat, G. C., M. Kim, L. L. Adams-Campbell, et al. (2009). Longitudinal study of serum carotenoid, retinol, and tocopherol concentrations in relation to breast cancer risk among postmenopausal women. *American Journal of Clinical Nutrition* 90 (1): 162–69.

Thomson, C. A., N. R. Stendell-Hollis, C. L. Rock, et al. (2007). Plasma and dietary carotenoids are associated with reduced oxidative stress in women previously treated for breast cancer. *Cancer Epidemiology, Biomarkers and Prevention* 16 (10): 2008–15.

Trejo-Solís, C., J. Pedraza-Chaverrí, M. Torres-Ramos, et al. (2013). Multiple molecular and cellular mechanisms of action of lycopene in cancer inhibition. *Evidence-Based Complementary and Alternative Medicine*, article ID 705121.

Yan, B., M. S. Lu, L. Wang, et al. (2016). Specific serum carotenoids are inversely associated with breast cancer risk among Chinese women: A case-control study. *British Journal of Nutrition* 15 (1): 129–37.

Hattori, M., K. Kawakami, M. Akimoto, et al. (2013). Antitumor effect of Japanese apricot extract (MK615) on human cancer cells in vitro and in vivo through a reactive oxygen species-dependent mechanism. *Tumori* 99 (2): 239–48.

BANANA

Bennett, R. N., T. M. Shiga, N. M. Hassimotto, et al. (2010). Phenolics and antioxidant properties of fruit pulp and cell wall fractions of postharvest banana (*Musa acuminate* Juss.) cultivars. *Journal of Agricultural and Food Chemistry* 58 (13): 7991–8003.

Kanazawa, K., and H. Sakakibara. (2000). High content of dopamine, a strong antioxidant, in Cavendish banana. *Journal of Agricultural and Food Chemistry* 48 (3): 844–48.

Sae-Teaw, M., J. Johns, N. P. Johns, et al. (2012). Serum melatonin levels and antioxidant capacities after consumption of pineapple, orange, or banana by healthy male volunteers. *Journal of Pineal Research* 55 (1): 58–64.

Slavin, J. (2013). Fiber and prebiotics: Mechanisms and health benefits. *Nutrients* 5 (4), 1417–35.

BASIL

Al-Ali, K. H., H. A. El-Beshbishy, et al. (2013). Cytotoxic activity of methanolic extract of *Mentha longifolia* and *Ocimum basilicum* against human breast cancer. *Pakistan Journal of Biological Sciences* 16 (23): 1744–50.

Huang, W. Y., Y. Z. Cai, and Y. Zhang. (2010). Natural phenolic compounds from medicinal herbs and dietary plants: Potential use for cancer prevention. *Nutrition and Cancer* 62 (1): 1–20.

Vidhya, N., and S. N. Devaraj. (2011). Induction of apoptosis by eugenol in human breast cancer cells. *Indian Journal of Experimental Biology* 49 (11): 871–78.

BEETS

Kabat, G. C., M. Kim, L. L. Adams-Campbell, et al. (2009). Longitudinal study of serum carotenoid, retinol, and tocopherol concentrations in relation to breast cancer risk among postmenopausal women. *American Journal of Clinical Nutrition* 90 (1): 162–69.

Tamimi, R. M., G. A. Colditz, and S. E. Hankinson. (2009). Circulating carotenoids, mammographic density, and subsequent risk of breast cancer. *Cancer Prevention Research* 69 (24): 9323–29.

BLACKBERRIES

Munagala, R., F. Aqil, M. V. Vadhanam, et al. (2013). MicroRNA "signature" during estrogen-mediated mammary carcinogenesis and its reversal by ellagic acid intervention. *Cancer Letters* 339 (2): 175–84.

Seeram, N. P., L. S. Adams, Y. Zhang, et al. (2006). Blackberry, black raspberry, blueberry, cranberry, red raspberry, and strawberry extracts inhibit growth and stimulate apoptosis of human cancer cells in vitro. *Journal of Agricultural and Food Chemistry* 54 (25): 9329–39.

BLACK PEPPER

Do, M. T., H. G. Kim, J. H. Choi, et al. (2013). Antitumor efficacy of piperine in the treatment of human HER2-overexpressing breast cancer cells. *Food Chemistry* 141 (3): 2591–99.

Doucette, C. D., A. L. Hilchie, R. Liwski, and D. W. Hoskin. (2012). Piperine, a dietary phytochemical, inhibits angiogenesis. *Journal of Nutritional Biochemistry* 24 (1): 231–39.

Majdalawieh, A. F., and R. I. Carr. (2010). In vitro investigation of the potential immunomodulatory and anticancer activities of black pepper (*Piper nigrum*) and cardamom (*Elettaria cardamomum*). *Journal of Medicinal Food* 13 (2): 371–81.

Sriwiriyajan, S., A. Tedasen, N. Lailerd, et al. (2016). Anticancer and cancer prevention effects of piperine-free *Piper nigrum* extract on N-nitrosomethylurea-induced mammary tumorigenesis in rats. *Cancer Prevention Research* 9 (1): 74–82.

BLACK RASPBERRIES

Seeram, N. P., L. S. Adams, Y. Zhang, et al. (2006). Blackberry, black raspberry, blueberry, cranberry, red raspberry, and strawberry extracts inhibit growth and stimulate apoptosis of human cancer cells in vitro. *Journal of Agricultural and Food Chemistry* 54 (25): 9329–39.

BLUEBERRIES

Adams, L. S., N. Kanaya, S. Phung, et al. (2011). Whole blueberry powder modulates the growth and metastasis of MDA-MB-231 triple negative breast tumors in mice. *Journal of Nutrition* 141 (10): 1805–12.

Adams, L. S., S. Phung, N. Yee, et al. (2010). Blueberry phytochemicals inhibit growth and metastatic potential of MDA-MB-231 breast cancer cells through modulation of the phosphatidylinositol 3-kinase pathway. *Cancer Research* 70 (9): 3594–605.

Fung, T. T., S. E. Chiuve, W. C. Willett, et al. (2013). Intake of specific fruits and vegetables in relation to risk of estrogen receptor–negative breast cancer among postmenopausal women. *Breast Cancer Treatment and Research* 138 (3): 925–30.

Mak, K. K., A. T. Wu, W. H. Lee, et al. (2013). Pterostilbene, a bioactive component of blueberries, suppresses the generation of breast cancer stem cells within tumor microenvironment and metastasis via modulating NF-κB/microR NA 448 circuit. *Molecular Nutrition and Food Research* 57 (7): 1123–34.

Olsson, M. E., K. E. Gustavsson, S. Andersson, et al. (2004). Inhibition of cancer cell proliferation in vitro by fruit and berry extracts and correlations with antioxidant levels. *Journal of Agricultural and Food Chemistry* 52 (24): 7264–71.

Ravoori, S., M. V. Vadhanam, F. Aqil, et al. (2012). Inhibition of estrogen-mediated mammary tumorigenesis by blueberry and black raspberry. *Journal of Agricultural and Food Chemistry* 60 (22): 5547–55.

Seeram, N. P., L. S. Adams, Y. Zhang, et al. (2006). Blackberry, black raspberry, blueberry, cranberry, red raspberry, and strawberry extracts inhibit growth and stimulate apoptosis of human cancer cells in vitro. *Journal of Agricultural and Food Chemistry* 54 (25): 9329–39.

CACHEXIA

Lopes de Campos-Ferraz, P. L., I. Andrade, W. das Neves, et al. (2014). An overview of amines as nutritional supplements to counteract cancer cachexia. *Journal of Cachexia, Sarcopenia and Muscle* 5 (2): 105–10.

CANTALOUPE

Eliassen, A. H., S. J. Hendrickson, L. A. Brinton, et al. (2012). Circulating carotenoids and risk of breast cancer: Pooled analysis of eight prospective studies. *Journal of the National Cancer Institute* 104 (24): 1905–16.

Kabat, G. C., M. Kim, L. L. Adams-Campbell, et al. (2009). Longitudinal study of serum carotenoid, retinol, and tocopherol concentrations in relation to breast cancer risk among postmenopausal women. *American Journal of Clinical Nutrition* 90 (1): 162–69.

Tamimi, R. M., G. A. Colditz, S. E. Hankinson, et al. (2009). Circulating carotenoids, mammographic density, and subsequent risk of breast cancer. *Cancer Research* 69 (24): 9323–29.

CARDAMOM

Acharya, A., I. Das, S. Singh, et al. (2010). Chemopreventive properties of indole-3-carbinol, diindolylmethane and other constituents of cardamom against carcinogenesis. *Recent Patents of Food, Nutrition and Agriculture* 2 (2): 166–77.

Majdalawieh, A. F., and R. I. Carr. (2010). In vitro investigation of the potential immunomodulatory and anticancer activities of black pepper (*Piper nigrum*) and cardamom (*Elettaria cardamomum*). *Journal of Medicinal Food* 13 (2): 371–81.

Marongiu, B., A. Piras, and S. Porcedda. (2004). Comparative analysis of the oil and supercritical CO^2 extract of Elettaria cardamomum (L.) Maton. *Journal of Agricultural and Food Chemistry* 52 (20): 6278–82.

Miller, J. A., J. E. Lang, M. Ley, et al. (2013). Human breast tissue disposition and bioactivity of limonene in women with early-stage breast cancer. *Cancer Prevention Research* 6 (6): 577–84.

CARROT

Larsson, S. C., L. Bergkvist, and A. Wolk. (2010). Dietary carotenoids and risk of hormone receptor-defined breast cancer in a prospective cohort of Swedish women. *European Journal of Cancer* 46 (6): 1079–85.

Mignone, L. I., E. Giovannucci, P. A. Newcomb, et al. (2009). Dietary carotenoids and the risk of invasive breast cancer. *International Journal of Cancer* 124 (12): 2929–37.

Rock, C. L., S. W. Flatt, L. Natarajan, et al. (2005). Plasma carotenoids and recurrence-free survival in women with a history of breast cancer. *Journal of Clinical Oncology* 23 (27): 6631–38.

Wang, Y., S. M. Gapstur, M. M. Gaudet, et al. (2015). Plasma carotenoids and breast cancer risk in the Cancer Prevention Study II Nutrition Cohort. *Cancer Causes & Control* 26 (9): 1233–44.

CHERRIES

Olsson, M. E., K. E. Gustavsson, S. Andersson, et al. (2004). Inhibition of cancer cell proliferation in vitro by fruit and berry extracts and correlations with antioxidant levels. *Journal of Agricultural and Food Chemistry* 52 (24): 7264–71.

CHIA SEED

Alfano, C. M., I. Imayama, M. L. Neuhouser, et al. (2012). Fatigue, inflammation, and ω-3 and ω-6 fatty acid intake among breast cancer survivors. *Journal of Clinical Oncology* 30 (12): 1280–87.

CILANTRO

Kabat, G. C., M. Kim, L. L. Adams-Campbell, et al. (2009). Longitudinal study of serum carotenoid, retinol, and tocopherol concentrations in relation to breast cancer risk among postmenopausal women. *American Journal of Clinical Nutrition* 90 (1): 162–69.

Tamimi, R. M., G. A. Colditz, and S. E. Hankinson. (2009). Circulating carotenoids, mammographic density, and subsequent risk of breast cancer. *Cancer Prevention Research* 69 (24): 9323–29.

CITRUS

Baek, S. H., S. M. Kim, D. Nam, et al. (2012). Antimetastatic effect of nobiletin through the down-regulation of CXC chemokine receptor type 4 and matrix metallopeptidase-9. *Pharmaceutical Biology* 50 (10): 1210–18.

Jabri Karoui, I., and B. Marzouk. (2013). Characterization of bioactive compounds in Tunisian bitter orange (*Citrus aurantium L.*) peel and juice and determination of their antioxidant activities. *BioMed Research International* 8 (1): 1–10.

Lee, C. J., L. Wilson, M. A. Jordan, et al. (2009). Hesperidin suppressed proliferations of both human breast cancer and androgen-dependent prostate cancer cells. *Phytotherapy Research* 24 Suppl 1: S15–19.

Li, H., B. Yang, J. Huang, et al. (2013). Naringin inhibits growth potential of human triple-negative breast cancer cells by targeting β-catenin signaling pathway. *Toxicology Letters* 220 (3): 219–28.

Miller, J. A., J. E. Lang, M. Ley, et al. (2013). Human breast tissue disposition and bioactivity of limonene in women with early-stage breast cancer. *Cancer Prevention Research* 6 (6): 577–84.

Tanaka, T., T. Tanaka, M. Tanaka, et al. (2011). Cancer chemoprevention by citrus pulp and juices containing high amounts of β-cryptoxanthin and hesperidin. *BioMed Research International* 2012:516981.

COCOA

Oleaga, C., M. García, A. Solé, et al. (2005). CYP1A1 is overexpressed upon incubation of breast cancer cells with a polyphenolic cocoa extract. *Molecular Cancer Therapeutics* 51 (4): 465–76.

Ramljak, D., L. J. Romanczyk, L. J. Metheny-Barlow, et al. (2005). Pentameric procyanidin from Theobroma cacao selectively inhibits growth of human breast cancer cells. *Molecular Cancer Therapeutics* 4 (4): 537–46.

CRANBERRIES

Duo, J., G. G. Ying, G. W. Wang, et al. (2012). Quercetin inhibits human breast cancer cell proliferation and induces apoptosis via Bcl-2 and Bax regulation. *Molecular Medicine Reports* 5 (6): 1453–56.

Munagala, R., F. Aqil, M. V. Vadhanam, et al. (2013). MicroRNA "signature" during estrogen-mediated mammary carcinogenesis and its reversal by ellagic acid intervention. *Cancer Letters* 339 (2): 175–84.

Seeram, N. P., L. S. Adams, Y. Zhang, et al. (2006). Blackberry, black raspberry, blueberry, cranberry, red raspberry, and strawberry extracts inhibit growth and stimulate apoptosis of human cancer cells in vitro. *Journal of Agricultural and Food Chemistry* 54 (25): 9329–39.

CULTURED COCONUT MILK

Maroof, H., Z. M. Hassan, A. M. Mobarez, et al. (2012). *Lactobacillus acidophilus* could modulate the immune response against breast cancer in murine model. *Journal of Clinical Immunology* 32 (6): 1353–59.

Tarko, T., A. Duda-Chodak, and N. Zajac. (2013). Digestion and absorption of phenolic compounds assessed by in vitro simulation methods. *Roczniki Państwowego Zakładu Higieny* 64 (2): 79–84.

GARLIC

Chandra-Kuntal, K., J. Lee, and S. V. Singh. (2013). Critical role for reactive oxygen species in apoptosis induction and cell migration inhibition by diallyl trisulfide, a cancer chemopreventive component of garlic. *Breast Cancer Treatment and Research* 138 (1): 69–79.

Galeone, C., C. Pelucchi, F. Levi, et al. (2006). Onion and garlic use and human cancer. *American Journal of Clinical Nutrition* 84 (5): 1027–32.

Milner, J. A. (2006). Preclinical Perspectives on Garlic and Cancer. *Journal of Nutrition* 136 (3 Suppl): 827S–831S.

Modem, S., S. E. Dicarlo, and T. R. Reddy. (2012). Fresh garlic extract induces growth arrest and morphological differentiation of MCF7 breast cancer cells. *Genes and Cancer* 3 (2): 177–86.

GINGER

Gan, F. F., H. Ling, X. Ang, et al. (2013). A novel shogaol analog suppresses cancer cell invasion and inflammation, and displays cytoprotective effects through modulation of NF-κB and Nrf2-Keap1 signaling pathways. *Toxicology and Applied Pharmacology* 272 (3): 852–62.

GRAPEFRUIT

Baek, S. H., S. M. Kim, D. Nam, et al. (2012). Antimetastatic effect of nobiletin through the down-regulation of CXC chemokine receptor type 4 and matrix metallopeptidase-9. *Pharmaceutical Biology* 50 (10): 1210–18.

Bhuvaneswari, V., and S. Nagini. (2005). Lycopene: A review of its potential as an anticancer agent. *Current Medicinal Therapy Anticancer Agents* 5 (6): 627–35.

Bulzomi, P., A. Bolli, P. Galluzzo, et al. (2012). The naringenin-induced proapoptotic effect in breast cancer cell lines holds out against a high bisphenol a background. *Journal of Nutrition* 64 (8): 690–96.

Lee, C. J., L. Wilson, M. A. Jordan, et al. (2009). Hesperidin suppressed proliferations of both human breast cancer and androgen-dependent prostate cancer cells. *Phytotherapy Research* 24 Suppl 1: S15–19.

GRAPES

Munagala, R., F. Aqil, M. V. Vadhanam, et al. (2013). MicroRNA "signature" during estrogen-mediated mammary carcinogenesis and its reversal by ellagic acid intervention. *Cancer Letters* 339 (2): 175–84.

Okic-Djordjevic, I., D. Trivanovic, J. Krstic, et al. (2013). GE132+Natural: Novel promising dietetic supplement with antiproliferative influence on prostate, colon, and breast cancer cells. *Journal of Balkan Union of Oncology* 18 (2): 504–10.

Sun, T., Q. Y. Chen, L. J. Wu, et al. (2012). Antitumor and antimetastatic activities of grape skin polyphenols in a murine model of breast cancer. *Food and Chemical Toxicology* 64 (9): 609–14.

GREENS

Eliassen, A. H., S. J. Hendrickson, L. A. Brinton, et al. (2012). Circulating carotenoids and risk of breast cancer: Pooled analysis of eight prospective studies. *Journal of the National Cancer Institute* 104 (24): 1905–16.

Eliassen, A. H., X. Liao, B. Rosner, et al. (2015). Plasma carotenoids and risk of breast cancer over 20 years of follow-up. *American Journal of Clinical Nutrition* 101 (6): 1197–205.

Emaus, M. J., P. H. Peeters, M. F. Bakker, et al. (2016). Vegetable and fruit consumption and the risk of hormone receptor-defined breast cancer in the EPIC cohort. *American Journal of Clinical Nutrition* 103 (1): 168–77.

Kabat, G. C., M. Kim, L. L. Adams-Campbell, et al. (2009). Longitudinal study of serum carotenoid, retinol, and tocopherol concentrations in relation to breast cancer risk among postmenopausal women. *American Journal of Clinical Nutrition* 90 (1): 162–69.

Yan, B., M. S. Lu, L. Wang, et al. (2016). Specific serum carotenoids are inversely associated with breast cancer risk among Chinese women: A case-control study. *British Journal of Nutrition* 115 (1): 129–37.

GREEN TEA

Braicu, C., C. D. Gherman, A. Irimie, et al. (2013). Epigallocatechin-gallate (EGCG) inhibits cell proliferation and migratory behavior of triple negative breast cancer cells. *Journal of Nanoscience and Nanotechnology* 13 (1): 632–37.

Donejko, M., M. Niczyporuk, E. Galicka, et al. (2013). Anticancer properties epigallo-catechin-gallate contained in green tea. *Postępy higieny i medycyny doświadczalnej* (Online) 67:26–34.

Gu, J. W., K. L. Makey, K. B. Tucker, et al. (2013). EGCG, a major green tea catechin suppresses breast tumor angiogenesis and growth via inhibiting the activation of HIF-1α and NFκB, and VEGF expression. *Vascular Cell* 5 (1): 9.

Yiannakopoulou, E. C. (2013). Effect of green tea catechins on breast carcinogenesis: A systematic review of in-vitro and in-vivo experimental studies. *European Journal of Cancer Prevention* 23 (2): 84–89.

Yiannakopoulou, E. C. (2013). Green tea catechins: Proposed mechanisms of action in breast cancer focusing on the interplay between survival and apoptosis. *Anticancer Agents Medicinal Chemistry* 14 (2): 290–95.

HEMPSEED

Jeong M, Cho J, Shin JI, Jeon YJ, Kim JH, Lee SJ, Kim ES, Lee K. (2016) Hempseed oil induces reactive oxygen species and C/EBP homologous protein-mediated apoptosis in MH7A human rheumatoid arthritis fibroblast–like synovial cells. *Journal of Ethnopharmacology.* 154 (3): 745–52.

HOLY BASIL

Nangia-Makker, P., T. Raz, L. Tait, et al. (2013). *Ocimum gratissimum* retards breast cancer growth and progression and is a natural inhibitor of matrix metalloproteases. *Cancer Biology and Therapy* 14 (5): 417–27.

KALE

Acharya, A., I. Das, S. Singh, et al. (2010). Chemopreventive properties of indole-3-carbinol, diindolylmethane and other constituents of cardamom against carcinogenesis. *Recent Patents of Food, Nutrition and Agriculture* 2 (2): 166–77.

Kabat, G. C., M. Kim, L. L. Adams-Campbell, et al. (2009). Longitudinal study of serum carotenoid, retinol, and tocopherol concentrations in relation to breast cancer risk among postmenopausal women. *American Journal of Clinical Nutrition* 90 (1): 162–69.

Tamimi, R. M., G. A. Colditz, and S. E. Hankinson. (2009). Circulating carotenoids, mammographic density, and subsequent risk of breast cancer. *Cancer Prevention Research* 69 (24): 9323–29.

LEMON

Baek, S. H., S. M. Kim, D. Nam, et al. (2012). Antimetastatic effect of nobiletin through the down-regulation of CXC chemokine receptor type 4 and matrix metallopeptidase-9. *Pharmaceutical Biology* 50 (10): 1210–18.

MANGO

Jordan, I., A. Hebestreit, B. Swai, et al. (2013). Dietary patterns and breast cancer risk among women in northern Tanzania: A case-control study. *European Journal of Nutrition* 52 (3): 905–15.

Matkowski, A., P. Kuśś, E. Góralska, et al. (2013). Mangiferin—a bioactive xanthonoid, not only from mango and not just antioxidant. *Mini Reviews in Medicinal Chemistry* 13 (3): 439–55.

OATS

Suzuki, R., A. C. M. Thiébaut, A. Fournier, et al. (2008). Dietary lignans and postmenopausal breast cancer risk by estrogen receptor status: A prospective cohort study of Swedish women. *British Journal of Cancer* 99 (6): 475–86.

Velentzis, L. S., M. M. Cantwell, C. Cardwell, et al. (2009). Lignans and breast cancer risk in pre- and post-menopausal women: Meta-analyses of observational studies. *British Journal of Cancer* 100 (9): 1492–98.

ORANGES

Baek, S. H., S. M. Kim, D. Nam, et al. (2012). Antimetastatic effect of nobiletin through the down-regulation of CXC chemokine receptor type 4 and matrix metallopeptidase-9. *Pharmaceutical Biology* 50 (10): 1210–18.

Lee, C. J., L. Wilson, M. A. Jordan, et al. (2009). Hesperidin suppressed proliferations of both human breast cancer and androgen-dependent prostate cancer cells. *Phytotherapy Research* 4 Suppl 1: S15–19.

Li, H., B. Yang, J. Huang, et al. (2013). Naringin inhibits growth potential of human triple-negative breast cancer cells by targeting β-catenin signaling pathway. *Toxicology Letters* 220 (3): 219–28.

ORGANIC

Baker, B. P., C. M. Benbrook, E. Groth III, et al. (2002). Pesticide residues in conventional, integrated pest management (IPM)-grown and organic foods: Insights from three US data sets. *Food Additives & Contaminants* 19 (5): 427–46.

Benbrook, C. (2013). Are organic foods safer or healthier? *Annals of Internal Medicine.* *http://www.eufic.org/.*

Benbrook, C. (2002). Organochlorine residues pose surprisingly high dietary risks. *Journal of the Epidemiology Community Health* 56 (11): 822–23.

PAPAYA

García-Solís, P., E. M. Yahia, V. Morales-Tlalpan, et al. (2009). Screening of antiproliferative effect of aqueous extracts of plant foods consumed in México on the breast cancer cell line MCF-7. *International Journal of Food Sciences and Nutrition* 60 Suppl 6: 32–46.

Rock, C. L., S. W. Flatt, L. Natarajan, et al. (2005). Plasma carotenoids and recurrence-free survival in women with a history of breast cancer. *Journal of Clinical Oncology* 23 (27): 6631–38.

PEACHES

Fung, T. T., S. E. Chiuve, W. C. Willett, et al. (2013). Intake of specific fruits and vegetables in relation to risk of estrogen receptor-negative breast cancer among postmenopausal women. *Breast Cancer Treatment and Research* 138 (3): 925–30.

Mignone, L. I., E. Giovannucci, P. A. Newcomb, et al. (2009). Dietary carotenoids and the risk of invasive breast cancer. *International Journal of Cancer* 124 (12): 2929–37.

Munagala, R., F. Aqil, M. V. Vadhanam, et al. (2013). MicroRNA "signature" during estrogen-mediated mammary carcinogenesis and its reversal by ellagic acid intervention. *Cancer Letters* 339 (2): 175–84.

Noratto, G., W. Porter, D. Byrne, et al. (2014). Polyphenolics from peach (*Prunus persica* var. Rich Lady) inhibit tumor growth and metastasis of MDA-MB-435 breast cancer cells in vivo. *Journal of Nutritional Biochemistry* 25 (7): 796–800.

PHYTOCHEMICALS

Sak, K. (2012). Chemotherapy and dietary phytochemical agents. *Chemotherapy Research and Practice*, article ID 282570.

PINEAPPLE

Bhui, K., S. Tyagi, B. Prakash, et al. (2010). Pineapple bromelain induces autophagy, facilitating apoptotic response in mammary carcinoma cells. *BioFactors* 36 (6): 474–82.

Dhandayuthapani, S., H. D. Perez, A. Paroulek, et al. (2012). Bromelain-induced apoptosis in GI-101A breast cancer cells. *Journal of Medicinal Food* 15 (4): 344–49.

PLUM

Ma, Z., L. Hou, Y. Jiang, et al. (2014). The endogenous oxindole isatin induces apoptosis of MCF-7 breast cancer cells through a mitochondrial pathway. *Oncology Report* 32 (5): 2111–17.

Radwan, A. A., F. K. Alanazi, and A. Al-Dhfyan. (2013). Synthesis, and docking studies of some fused-quinazolines and quinazolines carrying biological active isatin moiety as cell-cycle inhibitors of breast cancer cell lines. *Drug Research* 63 (3): 129–36.

Vizzotto, M., W. Porter, D. Byrne, et al. (2014). Polyphenols of selected peach and plum genotypes reduce cell viability and inhibit proliferation of breast cancer cells while not affecting normal cells. *Food Chemistry* 164:363–70.

Yu, M. H., H. G. Im, S. O. Lee, et al. (2007). Induction of apoptosis by immature fruits of *Prunus salicina* Lindl. cv. Soldam in MDA-MB-231 human breast cancer cells. *International Journal of Food Sciences and Nutrition* 58 (1): 42–53.

POMEGRANATE

Adhami, V. M., N. Khan, and H. Mukhtar. (2009). Cancer chemoprevention by pomegranate: Laboratory and clinical evidence. *Nutrition and Cancer* 61 (6): 811–15.

Kim, N. D., R. Mehta, W. Yu, et al. (2002). Chemopreventive and adjuvant therapeutic potential of pomegranate (*Punica granatum*) for human breast cancer. *Breast Cancer Treatment and Research* 71 (3): 203–17.

Munagala, R., F. Aqil, M. V. Vadhanam, et al. (2013). MicroRNA "signature" during estrogen-mediated mammary carcinogenesis and its reversal by ellagic acid intervention. *Cancer Letters* 339 (2): 175–84.

Rocha, A., L. Wang, M. Penichet, et al. (2012). Pomegranate juice and specific components inhibit cell and molecular processes critical for metastasis of breast cancer. *Breast Cancer Treatment and Research* 136 (3): 647–58.

Sreekumar, S., H. Sithul, P. Muraleedharan, et al. (2014). Pomegranate fruit as a rich source of biologically active compounds. *BioMed Research International*, article ID 686921.

Vini, R., and S. Sreeja. (2015). *Punica granatum* and its therapeutic implications on breast carcinogenesis: A review. *Biofactors* 41 (2): 78–89.

PROBIOTICS

Aragón, F., S. Carino, G. Perdigón, et al. (2014). The administration of milk fermented by the probiotic *Lactobacillus casei* CRL 431 exerts an immunomodulatory effect against a breast tumour in a mouse model. *Immunobiology* 219 (6): 457–64.

PRUNES

Yu, M. H., H.G. Im, S. O. Lee, et al. (2007). Induction of apoptosis by immature fruits of Prunus *salicina* Lindl. cv. Soldam in MDA-MB-231 human breast cancer cells. *International Journal of Food Sciences and Nutrition* 58 (1): 42–53.

RED RASPBERRIES

Munagala, R., F. Aqil, M. V. Vadhanam, et al. (2013). MicroRNA "signature" during estrogen-mediated mammary carcinogenesis and its reversal by ellagic acid intervention. *Cancer Letters* 339 (2): 175–84.

Olsson, M. E., K. E. Gustavsson, S. Andersson, et al. (2004). Inhibition of cancer cell proliferation in vitro by fruit and berry extracts and correlations with antioxidant levels. *Journal of Agricultural and Food Chemistry* 52 (24): 7264–71.

ROSEMARY

Berdowska, I., B. Zieliński, I. Fecka, et al. (2013). Cytotoxic impact of phenolics from Lamiaceae species on human breast cancer cells. *Food Chemistry* 41 (2): 1313–21.

Einbond, L. S., H. A. Wu, R. Kashiwazaki, et al. (2012). Carnosic acid inhibits the growth of ER-negative human breast cancer cells and synergizes with curcumin. *Fitoterapia* 83 (7): 1160–68.

Johnson, J. J. (2011). Carnosol: A promising anticancer and anti-inflammatory agent. *Cancer Letters* 305 (1): 1–7.

Ngo, S. N., D. B. Williams, and R. J. Head. (2011). Rosemary and cancer prevention: Preclinical perspectives. *Critical Reviews in Food Science and Nutrition* 51 (10): 946–54.

Yesil-Celiktas, O., C. Sevimli, E. Bedir, et al. (2010). Inhibitory effects of rosemary extracts, carnosic acid and rosmarinic acid on the growth of various human cancer cell lines. *Plant Foods and Human Nutrition* 65 (2): 158–63.

STRAWBERRIES

Munagala, R., F. Aqil, M. V. Vadhanam, et al. (2013). MicroRNA "signature" during estrogen-mediated mammary carcinogenesis and its reversal by ellagic acid intervention. *Cancer Letters* 339 (2): 175–84.

Seeram, N. P., L. S. Adams, Y. Zhang, et al. (2006). Blackberry, black raspberry, blueberry, cranberry, red raspberry, and strawberry extracts inhibit growth and stimulate apoptosis of human cancer cells in vitro. *Journal of Agricultural and Food Chemistry* 54 (25): 9329–39.

Somasagara, R. R., M. Hegde, K. K. Chiruvella, et al. (2012). Extracts of strawberry fruits induce intrinsic pathway of apoptosis in breast cancer cells and inhibits tumor progression in mice. *PLoS One* 7 (10): e47021.

SUBTYPES

Shivappa, N., S. Sandin, M. Löf, et al. (2015). Prospective study of dietary inflammatory index and risk of breast cancer in Swedish women. *British Journal of Cancer*
113 (7): 1099–103.

Tin, A. S., A. H. Park, S. N. Sundar, et al. (2014). Essential role of the cancer stem/
progenitor cell marker nucleostemin for indole-3-carbinol anti-proliferative
responsiveness in human breast cancer cells. *BMC Biology* 12:72.

SUNFLOWER SEEDS

Suzuki, R., T. Rylander-Rudqvist, S. Saji, et al. (2008). Dietary lignans and postmenopausal breast cancer risk by estrogen receptor status: A prospective cohort study
of Swedish women. *British Journal of Cancer* 98 (3): 636–40.

SYNERGISTIC EFFECTS

Liu, R. H. (2003). Health benefits of fruit and vegetables are from additive and synergistic combinations of phytochemicals. *American Society for Clinical Nutrition*
78 (3): 517S–520S.

TANGERINES

Baek, S. H., S. M. Kim, D. Nam, et al. (2012). Antimetastatic effect of nobiletin through
the down-regulation of CXC chemokine receptor type 4 and matrix metallopepti-
dase-9. *Pharmaceutical Biology* 50 (10): 1210–18.

Lee, C. J., L. Wilson, M. A. Jordan, et al. (2009). Hesperidin suppressed proliferations of both human breast cancer and androgen-dependent prostate cancer cells.
Phytotherapy Research 24 Suppl 1: S15–19.

Lopez-Carillo, L., R. U. Hernandez-Ramirez, A. M. Calafat, et al. (2010). Exposure
to phthalates and breast cancer risk in Northern Mexico. *Environmental Health*
118 (4): 539–44.

TART CHERRIES

Martin, K. R., and A. Wooden. (2012). Tart cherry juice induces differential dose-dependent effects on apoptosis, but not cellular proliferation, in MCF-7 human breast cancer cells. *Journal of Medicinal Food* 15 (11): 945–54.

TOMATO

Bhuvaneswari, V., and S. Nagini. (2005). Lycopene: A review of its potential as an anticancer agent. *Current Medicinal Therapy Anticancer Agents* 5 (6): 627–35.

Mignone, L. I., E. Giovannucci, P. A. Newcomb, et al. (2009). Dietary carotenoids and the risk of invasive breast cancer. *International Journal of Cancer* 124 (12): 2929–37.

Thomson, C. A., N. R. Stendell-Hollis, C. L. Rock, et al. (2007). Plasma and dietary carotenoids are associated with reduced oxidative stress in women previously treated for breast cancer. *Cancer Epidemiology Biomarkers and Prevention* 16 (10): 2008–15.

Yan, B., M. S. Lu, L. Wang, et al. (2016). Specific serum carotenoids are inversely associated with breast cancer risk among Chinese women: A case-control study. *British Journal of Nutrition* 15 (1): 129–37.

TURMERIC

Alfano, C. M., I. Imayama, M. L. Neuhouser, et al. (2012). Fatigue, inflammation, and ω-3 and ω-6 fatty acid intake among breast cancer survivors. *Journal of Clinical Oncology* 30 (12): 1280–87.

Xia, Y., L. Jin, B. Zhang, et al. (2007). The potentiation of curcumin on insulin-like growth factor-1 action in MCF-7 human breast carcinoma cells. *Life Sciences* 80 (23): 2161–69.

VANILLA

Lirdprapamongkol, K., H. Sakurai, N. Kawasaki, et al. (2005). Vanillin suppresses in vitro invasion and in vivo metastasis of mouse breast cancer cells. *European Journal of Pharmaceutical Sciences* 25 (1): 57–65.

Shi, Z. Y., Y. Q. Li, Y. H. Kang, et al. (2012). Piperonal ciprofloxacin hydrazone induces growth arrest and apoptosis of human hepatocarcinoma SMMC-7721 cells. *Journal of the Chinese Pharmacological Society* 33 (2): 271–78.

WATERMELON

Bhuvaneswari, V., and S. Nagini. (2005). Lycopene: A review of its potential as an anticancer agent. *Current Medicinal Chemistry Anticancer Agents* 5 (6): 627–35.

Mignone, L. I., E. Giovannucci, P. A. Newcomb, et al. (2009). Dietary carotenoids and the risk of invasive breast cancer. *International Journal of Cancer* 124 (12): 2929–37.

WILD BLUEBERRIES

Dinstel, R. R., J. Cascio, and S. Koukel. (2013). The antioxidant level of Alaska's wild berries: High, higher and highest. *International Journal of Circumpolar Health* (August 5): 72.

GLOSSARY OF TERMS

The glossary contains medical, nutrition, and technical terms used in the explanations of the health benefits of food nutrients. Medical terminology is included, as these terms have specific biological meaning and accurately convey the results of studies and the activity of specific food nutrients. The following definitions cover a few of the most commonly used terms throughout the book.

Adjuvant: often refers to a substance or treatment used in conjunction with the initial or primary cancer treatment.

Alpha-carotene: part of the carotenoid family, carotenes are nutrients that are synthesized by plants. Animals (including humans) cannot make them and so have to eat plants to get them. Carotenes, the name of which is derived from carrots, are responsible for the orange color of carrots, sweet potatoes, and other plants. Alpha-carotene is a precursor of vitamin A and a strong antioxidant. Higher blood levels of alpha-carotene are associated with a lower incidence of mortality from breast cancer.

Angiogenesis: the growth of new blood vessels from preexisting blood vessels that supply cells or benign (harmless) tumors with blood and nutrients for growth, which may then become malignant (cancerous). Without a blood supply, cancers can't grow.

Anthocyanin: particularly powerful phytonutrients, anthocyanins from peaches and plums reduce cell proliferation in estrogen-dependent breast cancer cells. *See* Flavonoid.

Anti-angiogenesis: a cancer therapy that interferes with the growth of new blood vessels, in particular, those feeding tumors. Currently researchers are studying the effects of certain foods, including blueberries, garlic, and green tea, for their anti-angiogenesis effects.

Anticancer: means "against cancer." A food, medication, or treatment that is termed "anticancer" is one that fights cancer, whether by selective destruction of cancer cells or by enhancing an organism's natural defenses against cancer.

Anti-inflammatory: the ability to reduce inflammation. Anti (against) and inflammatory (inflammation causing) is a term used for a substance, such as a food, nutrient, or medication, that reduces inflammation.

Antioxidant: a substance that acts as a scavenger of free radicals, thus lessening or preventing oxidation (*see* Oxidation). Oxidative stress can lead to genetic damage that triggers cancer. *See also* Phenols and Flavonoids.

Antiproliferative: used to describe the reduction of growth and spread of cancer cells.

Antitumor: reduces the occurrence, severity, or risk of tumors.

Apoptosis: the programmed destruction of cells, which allows cancer cells to kill themselves without adversely affecting normal cells.

Autophagy: cell degradation by self-destruction. Food nutrients can trigger this reaction. For example, pineapple, which contains an enzyme called bromelain, has been shown to trigger autophagy of breast cancer cells.

Beta-carotenes: red-orange, fat-soluble nutrients that are converted to vitamin A in the body.

Bioactive: biological activity that describes either the beneficial or adverse effects of a substance on living matter. This term has traditionally been applied to pharmacological activity, but it can also be used to describe the effects of a nutrient or toxin on living matter.

Biomarker: short for biological marker, something that can be measured to assess a biological state or health status.

Bisphenol A (BPA): a manmade substance used to manufacture plastics; linked to an increased risk of breast cancer and other cancers.

Carcinogenic: capable of causing cancer.

Carotenes: nutrients from plants that have antioxidant properties. *See* Carotenoids.

Carotenoids: broadly classified into two classes, carotenes (alpha-carotene, beta-carotene, and lycopene) and xanthophylls (beta-cryptoxanthin, lutein, and zeaxanthin). Alpha-carotene, beta-carotene, and beta-cryptoxanthin are provitamin A carotenoids, meaning they can be converted by the body to retinol, a form of vitamin A. Carotenoids also have antioxidant properties.

Catechins: nutrients found in tea, cocoa, and some fruits and vegetables, such as epigallocatechin-gallate (EGCG), that reduce the potential for environmental toxins to act as carcinogens.

Cell cycle: the process by which cells are created, grow, and die. In cancer, the cell cycle is abnormal. Cells divide to form new cells much more quickly than in normal tissue. The extra cells build up and form tumors.

Cell markers: biochemical or genetic attributes that are different for different types of cells.

Cell migration: movement of a group of cells from one place to another.

Cell proliferation: increase in the number of cells or growth in a certain cell type.

Chemopreventive: the use of chemical agents, drugs, or food nutrients to prevent the development of cancer.

Cohort study: an observational study that follows a population who do not have a particular disease, while comparing their life histories with people who have the disease. Usually performed to identify risk factors.

Docosahexaenoic acid (DHA): a fatty acid, primarily found in nuts and seeds, that is extracted from algae and sold in supplements that may help increase the effect of chemotherapy on cancer cells.

Dopamine: a hormone that acts as a neurotransmitter.

Ellagic acid: a phenol found in fruits and vegetables that has antiproliferative and antioxidant properties.

Epigallocatechin-gallate (EGCG): an antioxidant found in green tea that inhibits cancer development and reduces cell proliferation in existing tumors via an epigenetic effect.

Estrogen receptor: a protein molecule within a cell that will only bind to estrogen or an estrogen analog. Once estrogen binds to the receptor, it can signal changes in the cell.

Fiber: the part of plant foods that acts as a prebiotic, feeding healthy gut microbes. Both soluble and insoluble forms of fiber bind with toxins, increase cellular receptivity to insulin, and hold moisture in the intestines, which improves hydration.

Flavonoids: nutrients from plants that have antioxidant, antibacterial, and anti-inflammatory properties. Isoflavonoids are a form of flavonoid.

Flavonols: flavonoids (including isoflavones) that inhibit breast carcinogenesis. They are found in plant foods such as onion, kale, broccoli, lettuce, tomatoes, apples, grapes, berries, and tea.

Free radical: an atom, molecule, or ion that has a "dangling" (unattached) covalent bond. This makes it prone to binding to other atoms or molecules.

When it binds to certain molecules within a cell, it can disrupt normal cell processes.

Genetically modified organism (GMO): a life form that has had a change deliberately induced in its genetic makeup. *See* Mutation.

Herbicides: compounds that kill weeds and other unwanted plants. These chemicals are often toxic and many are classified as carcinogens.

Hesperidin: flavonoid found in citrus fruits that may be particularly effective in preventing hormone-related cancers by interrupting hormone receptor binding in cancerous cells.

High mammographic density: an area of dense breast tissue that shows up on a mammogram.

Hormones: chemical messengers made by the body and released into the blood where they are carried to other parts of the body.

Hormone sensitive: Some tumors are made up of cells with specific hormone receptors. For example, if the cells react to estrogen, they are termed ER+ (estrogen receptor positive) or PR+ (progesterone receptor positive). If they do not respond to these hormones, they are termed accordingly, such as ER- (estrogen receptor negative). Cells that are hormone sensitive depend on hormones for stimulation and growth.

Immune system: the body's defense system against disease.

Incidence: the rate at which something occurs; for example, the incidence of breast cancer in women over fifty.

Indole-3-carbinol: nutrient found in brassica vegetables that may have anti-carcinogenic effects.

Inflammation: the body's physical response to stress, such as injury or infection, which can include pain, swelling, redness, and loss of function. While inflammation is a normal part of the immune system response to an acute injury or illness, chronic inflammation can cause permanent damage.

Insulin-like growth factor (IGF): substance secreted by the liver that limits cell death (apoptosis). May play a role in stimulating breast cancer growth.

Laboratory studies: any study done in a laboratory; usually refers to in vitro studies, but some in vivo studies are also laboratory studies. Studies done in a laboratory can usually be strictly controlled so that unexpected variables do not affect the study.

Lignans and enterolignans: fibrous plant compounds that have antioxidant, anti-inflammatory, and anticancer properties. Lignans are especially important for those with hormone-sensitive breast cancer as they are structurally similar to estrogen and can bind to estrogen receptors, thus blocking the actions of estrogen in the body.

Limonene: a compound found in the peels of lemons and other citrus fruits that has epigenetic and anti-angiogenesis properties.

Lutein: a xanthophyll carotenoid found in green leafy vegetables, eggs, and animal fat that provides protection against benign breast disease (BBD), an independent risk factor for breast cancer, through antioxidative or anti-proliferative mechanisms.

Lycopene: a carotenoid with the capacity to affect breast cancer as it inhibits cell proliferation, arrests the cell cycle in different phases, and increases apoptosis.

Melatonin: a hormone that helps regulate the sleep cycle; also has anti-inflammatory properties. Dysregulation of melatonin is believed to be a causative factor in breast cancer development for night workers, insomniacs, and those who suffer from chronic interrupted sleep.

Metabolism: the chemical reactions within the body that sustain life. Metabolism comprises two functions: catabolism (breakdown of components) and anabolism (creation of new components).

Metabolites: substances that result from catabolism of components. Estrogen metabolites, for example, result from the breakdown of the hormone estrogen.

Mutagenic: capable of causing changes in DNA that lead to mutations.

Mutation: a change in a gene that causes an organism to develop in a different way. Many mutations are spontaneous: they happen for reasons not yet understood. Mutation can also be induced, usually by chemicals or radiation. *See* GMO.

Naringenin: a flavonoid found in citrus fruits and tomatoes that may have protective effects against damage from BPA and also promote apoptosis in cancer cells. It may be effective in the treatment of triple-negative breast cancer.

Nobiletin: a flavonoid found in citrus fruits and in concentrated amounts in citrus fruit peels. The most-studied properties of nobiletin are its anti-inflammatory, cholesterol-lowering, and anticancer activities. Nobiletin may have the potential to suppress metastasis of breast cancer.

Omega-3 fatty acids: polyunsaturated fatty acids found in whole foods such as flaxseed, chia seed, and avocados. These essential fats inhibit cell proliferation and induce apoptosis in human breast cancer cells, especially the triple-negative subtype.

Omega-6 fatty acids: polyunsaturated fatty acids found in corn, soybeans, rapeseed, sunflower oils, and many other foods. A diet higher in omega-6 fatty acids and lower in omega-3 fatty acids may have negative health effects.

Oncology: medical specialty that studies and treats cancer. Cancer specialists are called oncologists.

Oxidation: a chemical reaction in cells that creates free radicals (*see* Free radical). Free radicals can trigger damaging changes in cells and even cause cell death. Cellular oxidation is a biological precursor to many cancers.

Oxidative stress: when the damage done by oxidation is greater than the body's ability to repair it.

Pesticides: compounds, generally chemically derived, that kill pests such as insects.

Phenols and polyphenols: phenols, polyphenols, and phenolics have anti-oxidant effects. Breast cancer survivors have a lower recurrence rate when their diets are rich in polyphenols from foods, such as broccoli, turmeric, pomegranate, and green tea.

Phytochemical: a chemical made by a plant. Anticancer phytochemicals include cyanidin, delphinidin, quercetin, kaempferol, ellagic acid, resveratrol, and pterostilbene.

Phytoestrogens: plant compounds that are structurally similar to the human hormone estrogen, which allows them to bind to sites on cells called estrogen receptors. They block estrogen from binding to the cells, which appears to reduce the chance of estrogen-stimulated cancer development.

Plasma: usually, the yellow fluid component of blood that cells float in. Can also refer to the fluid in or around cells.

Postmenopausal: after menopause is complete.

Prebiotics: dietary fiber that may enhance growth of helpful bacteria in the lower digestive tract.

Premenopausal: the period leading up to menopause. Some women have noticeable emotional swings, changes in periods, and other physical changes for one or more years before menopause.

Probiotics: microorganisms from food or supplements that help restore a healthy balance of bacteria in the intestines.

Procyanidins: a type of flavonoid.

Quercetin: a phytoestrogen that can block estrogen from binding to estrogen receptor beta sites, protecting against the development of estrogen-stimulated cancer. Quercetin also helps mitigate the toxic effects of BPA, a known breast toxin.

Recurrence: relapse, as when a cancer comes back after remission.

Shogaol: active compound formed from the gingerol in fresh and dried ginger that is responsible for ginger's antinausea, antidiarrheal, and apoptotic effects.

Signaling pathway: the chain of events that follows from a certain signal being given to a cell.

Significant association: a statistical term meaning that two or more things have been shown to be related in a way that is more than just chance. For instance, smoking tobacco has been shown to have a significant association with lung cancer.

Synergistic effect: when two or more things combine to have a greater effect than would be expected as a result of each separate thing.

Tangeretin: flavone found in the peels of tangerines and other citrus fruits; known to trigger apoptosis in human breast cancer cells.

Triple-negative breast cancers: also known as TNBC, a group of cancers that are not hormone modified.

ACKNOWLEDGMENTS

For Jennifer Lomax, my client and friend. Thank you for sharing your healing milestones and experiences as you navigated breast cancer and ultimately your triumphant return to your athletic self.

My deepest gratitude to Linda Konner, Allison Janse, Olivia Brent, McKenzie Johnson, Patrick Jennings, Kim Weiss, Taylor Grossman, Dr. Neal Barnard, Lise Alschuler, Linda Landkammer, Andrea Knutsen, Helen Gray, Jack Pokorny, Sophie Elan, Anne Rierson, Cassidy Stockton, and Karie Duff.

RESOURCES

Visit *DaniellaChace.com* for articles, recipes, and news about breast cancer research.

Where to Find and Order Products

Buy organic produce at your local farmer's market, co-op, or grocery store. If you can't find what you need there, you may be able to order it from *amazon.com* or other online sources. These are a few of the companies that I purchase smoothie ingredients from regularly.

Bob's Red Mill
bobsredmill.com

Bob's Red Mill Natural Foods offers a wide selection of natural and organic products, such as gluten-free oats, sunflower seeds, and chia and hemp seeds.

Frontier Natural Products Co-op
frontiercoop.com

Frontier products can be found in the bulk section of many grocery stores, food co-ops, and online. Frontier is a premier supplier of more than four hundred products, including herbs and spices such as turmeric powder, dried basil leaves, dried tulsi (holy basil), green tea, cinnamon, vanilla beans, vanilla extract, peppercorns, and chia seed.

Mighty Nest

mightynest.com

MightyNest is a website that provides advice about toxins and home products. You can order natural, organic, and nontoxic products all in one place. All of their products are free from known toxic ingredients, such as BPA, PVC, phthalates, lead, melamine, formaldehyde, flame retardants, parabens, and more. Their company mission: "Our dream is for MightyNest to become a place where people feel motivated and empowered, not discouraged and judged; somewhere people feel encouraged to make changes in their lives, whether large or small. We truly believe that simple changes bring mighty impact."

Further Reading

The Definitive Guide to Cancer: An Integrative Approach to Prevention, Treatment, and Healing. By Lise Alschuler and Karolyn A. Gazella. 3rd ed. (Celestial Arts, 2010).

The Definitive Guide to Thriving After Cancer: A Five-Step Integrative Plan to Reduce the Risk of Recurrence and Build Lifelong Health. By Lise Alschuler and Karolyn A. Gazella (Ten Speed Press, 2013).

Turning Off Breast Cancer: A Personalized Approach to Nutrition and Detoxification in Prevention and Healing. By Daniella Chace (Skyhorse Publishing, 2015).

ABOUT THE AUTHOR

Daniella Chace, MS, CN, is a clinical nutritionist and educator. She is an expert in personalized medical nutrition therapy, with an emphasis in toxicology, epigenetics, human microbial ecology, and orthomolecular applications in disease management. She is the author of more than twenty nutrition books and the host of NPR's *Nutrition Matters*. She lives in Port Townsend, Washington, where she sees clients in her private practice and develops recipes that support healing. Learn more at *daniellachace.com*.

Ms. Chace is the author and coauthor of numerous health and nutrition books including:

Superfood Smoothie Bowls: Delicious, Satisfying, Protein-Packed Blends that Boost Energy and Burn Fat (Running Press, 2017).

Healing Smoothies: 100 Research-Based, Delicious Recipes that Provide Nutrition Support for Cancer Prevention and Recovery (Skyhorse Press, 2015).

Turning Off Breast Cancer: A Personalized Approach to Nutrition and Detoxification in Prevention and Healing (Skyhorse Press, 2015).

*365 Skinny Smoothies: Delicious Recipes to Help You
Get Slim and Stay Healthy Every Day of the Year*
(Harlequin Nonfiction, 2014).

*The Detox Diet: The Definitive Guide for Lifelong Vitality
with Recipes, Menus, and Detox Plans,* with Dr. Elson M. Haas. 3rd ed.
(Ten Speed Press, 2012).

More Smoothies for Life: Satisfy, Energize and Heal Your Body
(Clarkson Potter, 2007).

*What to Eat if You Have Cancer: Healing Foods that Boost
Your Immune System*, with Maureen Keane. Updated 2nd ed.
(McGraw-Hill, 2006).

*What to Eat if You Have Diabetes: Healing Foods that Boost
Your Immune System*, with Maureen Keane. Updated 2nd ed.
(McGraw-Hill, 2005).

*The New Detox Diet: The Complete Guide for Lifelong Vitality
with Recipes, Menus, and Detox Plans*, with Dr. Elson Haas
(Celestial Arts, 2004).

Smoothies for Life! Yummy, Fun, and Nutritious!
(Clarkson Potter, 1998).

INDEX

From Patients and
Medical Professionals . . .

"This book is really great! I have already tried a bunch of the smoothies, and they are delicious. Having assembled my favorite fruits and the other ingredients Daniella recommends, it is easy to start off each day with one of these. I look forward to it. I also appreciate the technical information contained in the medical research Daniella has ferreted out, so I can use these recipes with total confidence in their healing properties."

—**Eileen R.**

"This book is a powerhouse of a resource—I love the author's time-saving tips and the explanation of nutritional science behind the ingredients. The recipes are easy—just a few ingredients—and delicious, and they are organized brilliantly. I have been making daily smoothies since I got the book, and it feels great to know I am nourishing my body with cancer-fighting yumminess. I am recommending it to all my friends."

—**Kimberly**

"Daniella Chace has done it yet once more. She is the most incredible nutritionist I have ever met. Being one of her clients myself, I can say that she transformed me and I will never look at nutrition the same way again. Right now I am getting back on track only due to her. Before I had even met Daniella she helped my mother battle cancer with her book *What to Eat When You Have Cancer*. I don't think my mother would have made it as well as she did without Daniella's nutrition guidance. Thank you, Daniella, for your incredible books—including this one."

—**Alysson Heazel**

"This new book by Daniella Chace masterfully delivers an easy-to-use, step-by-step guide, to create nutritional meals for anyone facing breast cancer. Each recipe is clearly and simply formatted to allow the reader to quickly assess what smoothie might best suit one's taste of the moment and/or specific nutritional needs. Each recipe also includes scientific research to both assure the reader of its efficacy as well as providing a link to the most up-to-date science on the subject of breast cancer. This book will surely become a 'treasured friend' as it is a compact gem of practical information. I will buy this book for anyone I know who is facing breast cancer."

—Jeanne Allen

"I would recommend this for anyone and everyone. Living with breast cancer all around me, it gives me some reassurance to know there is something more I can do to help my body's fight against this. I am telling everyone about this one!"

—Julie Mermelstein

"Having gluten, sugar, and dairy intolerance, I drink smoothies on a daily basis, so I was delighted to learn so much more about the disease prevention qualities of the ingredients incorporated in these recipes. I am giving my smoothie regime a bit of a healthy overhaul based on Daniella's recommendations! This book is useful for anyone who is interested in achieving better overall wellness. Parents should be raising their children with this type of dietary foundation! Daniella's research should prove to be invaluable and even life saving for many people, so I am grateful for her extensive time commitment towards helping others achieve better health."

—Sara Patterson

"In 2002, when I was diagnosed with breast cancer, there were few alternatives for treatment after surgery other than radiation and chemo. When Daniella invited my husband and I to taste test some of the recipes in *Breast*

Cancer Smoothies, I was excited to be a part of a support for prevention and recovery of cancer. Having taste tested some of the smoothies in this book I can say that they are tasty and go down easy. This is a book well worth exploring and using!"

—Helen Hesketh,
breast cancer survivor

"Finally a resource that matches cutting-edge research with easy-to-make recipes. This handy book offers a clear and efficient strategy for staying well or returning to wellness after a cancer diagnosis. Smoothies fit conveniently into any lifestyle and pack a lot of nutritional punch while limiting calories and eliminating artificial ingredients. These daily smoothies will retrain the palette to appreciate the wholesome goodness of whole foods that our bodies crave. The artificial flavors, sweeteners, fats and byproducts of processed foods will lose their bling when compared with the richness of real food. Empowered with the data-driven recipes included in *Breast Cancer Smoothies*, we can reclaim our wellness for a happier, healthier world."

—Jennifer Lomax

"In this book, Daniella provides over 100 smoothie recipes that can have a profound effect on breast cancer. From herbs to vegetables to fruits, the common thread is that these natural substances are chock full of phytonutrients, anticancer compounds, and antioxidants. In recipe after recipe, Daniella shows how proper nutrition can have an epigenetic effect and is essential in both preventing and treating breast cancer. She not only describes the ingredients and shows you how to make the tastiest smoothies you've ever tried, but she also cites the studies to prove their health effects. Use this book as you 'smoothie' your way to optimal health. You'll be glad you did."

—Ty M. Bollinger,
author and documentary film producer

"Better nutrition recipe books are important guides for patients and consumers seeking to improve their health and treatment programs. Chace has devoted much of her nutritional writing about the use and preparation of smoothies that offer both superb taste and science-based recipes. It is rare, indeed, for one to understand the cancer-fighting characteristics as documented in journal articles while preparing a smoothie. Equally impressive is the passionate description of her smoothies, reminding one of the wine connoisseur's appraisal of a particular vintage. Chace's book not only is a useful mixing guide but an up-to-date reference for those needing to study the anticancer activity of foods. Bravo to Chace!"

—Jonathan Collin, MD,
publisher of the *Townsend Letter*

"Nutrition is an absolute key to both preventing and recovering from breast cancer. Daniella has incorporated delicious, easy-to-follow smoothie recipes that are a perfect vehicle to deliver powerful anticancer phytochemicals that can really make a difference. The information is provided in an engaging format that is both practical and informative."

—**Michael T. Murray, N.D.**, coauthor,
How to Prevent and Treat Cancer with Natural Medicine